W9-CCN-281

# Seizures and Epilepsy
# in Childhood:
# A Guide for Parents

**Dr. John M. Freeman** is Lederer Professor of Pediatric Epilepsy and Director of the Pediatric Epilepsy Center at the Johns Hopkins Medical Institutions. He is also a vice-president of the Epilepsy Foundation of America and member of the Professional Advisory Board of the Epilepsy Foundation of America.

**Dr. Eileen P. G. Vining** is Associate Professor of Neurology and Pediatrics and Deputy Director of the Pediatric Epilepsy Center at the Johns Hopkins Medical Institutions. She is chairman of the Client and Public Affairs Committee of the Professional Advisory Board of the Epilepsy Foundation of America.

**Ms. Diana J. Pillas** is the Coordinator-Counselor of the Pediatric Epilepsy Center at the Johns Hopkins Medical Institutions and former president of the Epilepsy Association of Maryland. She is a vice-president of the Epilepsy Foundation of America and chairman of the Affiliate Affairs Committee of the Epilepsy Foundation of America.

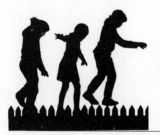

# Seizures and Epilepsy in Childhood: A Guide for Parents

**John M. Freeman, M.D.**
**Eileen P. G. Vining, M.D.**
**Diana J. Pillas**

The Pediatric Epilepsy Center
The Johns Hopkins Medical Institutions
Baltimore, Maryland

**The Johns Hopkins University Press**
**Baltimore and London**

© 1990 The Johns Hopkins University Press
All rights reserved. Published 1990
Printed in the United States of America on acid-free paper

Second printing, 1991
Johns Hopkins Paperbacks edition, 1993
Second printing, paperback, 1993

Illustrations in chapters 1, 6, and 9 by Timothy H. Phelps,
M.S., F.A.M.I.

The Johns Hopkins University Press
2715 North Charles Street
Baltimore, Maryland 21218-4319
The Johns Hopkins Press Ltd., London

Library of Congress Cataloging-in-Publication Data
Freeman, John Mark
   Seizures and epilepsy in childhood : a guide for parents
/John M. Freeman, Eileen P. G. Vining, Diana J. Pillas.
      p.     cm.
   Includes index.
   ISBN 0-8018-4049-X (alk. paper)   ISBN 0-8018-4649-8 (pbk.)
   1. Epilepsy in children—Popular works. 2. Convulsions
in children—Popular works. I. Vining, Eileen P. G.,
date   . II. Pillas, Diana, J., date   . III. Title.
RJ496.E6F7  1990
618.92'853—dc20                                90-4616 CIP


A catalog record for this book is available from the British Library.

To Dr. Horace Hodes,
Dr. David B. Clark,
Dr. Mary Betty Stevens
*We hope that we have a similar influence*
*on our own students.*

# Note to the Reader

This book embodies our approach to seizures and epilepsy *in general*. It was not written about *your* child. While we believe and practice its philosophy, we adjust our approach to suit each child's particular need and each family's situation. Obviously we would not treat your child without first learning a great deal about him or her, and so your child's treatment should not be based solely on what is written here. It must be developed in a dialogue between you and your child's physician. Our book is written to help you with that dialogue.

John M. Freeman, M.D.
Eileen P. G. Vining, M.D.
Diana J. Pillas

# Contents

## Part Four
## Coping with Epilepsy

# Illustrations

# Tables

# Foreword

by Tony Coelho, *Former Congressman from California,*
*Vice-President of the Epilepsy Foundation of America*

---

Being a parent is a wonderful experience that is full of challenges. We share in our child's joy over each accomplishment and we hurt—sometimes even more than our child—over the frustrations and challenges of growing up. During emotionally challenging times, children look to their parents not only for empathy and understanding but, more importantly, for strength. The purpose of this book is to equip parents with knowledge and strength to help their children meet, tackle, and control the challenges of epilepsy.

I have a special interest in this subject, because I have epilepsy. When I first started having seizures, almost thirty years ago, my parents did not have the resources to learn the truth about this disorder. My condition went undiagnosed and untreated for several years, but, thankfully, my seizures were infrequent enough to allow me to enjoy a college career. It was only after graduation, as I prepared to enter the Catholic priesthood, that my epilepsy was diagnosed and that I first encountered the stigma of being labeled an "epileptic." As I reeled from the disappointments of being denied admission to the seminary, losing my driver's license, and not being able to find a job, my parents were sharing in my hurt. But because epilepsy was misunderstood, they could not provide me with the strength I so desperately needed during that critical time.

Happily, both the field of medicine and the public perception of epilepsy have changed dramatically since I was a child. There are now excellent resources for people with epilepsy, and Johns Hopkins has pulled together the best of the best in this comprehensive guide.

As a parent, you know that epilepsy poses a challenge for you and your child. Many boundaries, however, are due to self-imposed limits and are not caused by epilepsy. As I learned about the disorder, I realized that the list of things I *could* do was infinitely longer than the list of things I could not do. Once that fact was realized, I decided that there were very few limits brought about by my epilepsy. I went on to pursue a career, was elected to Congress, and am now tackling a new challenge in the field of investment banking.

Mine is an epilepsy success story because of many circumstances for which I am grateful. But I am not the exception, for every day parents and children work together to face the challenges of epilepsy. With resources such as this book, parents will be well prepared to face this challenge and provide their children with love, strength, and the knowledge they need to live a full life.

# Preface

"It was the most frightening experience of our lives. We heard a noise; I guess it woke us up. We rushed into Caroline's bedroom, and there she was—choking, thrashing around. We thought she was going to die. We'd never seen a seizure and didn't know what it was. By the time the ambulance arrived, the seizure was over and she was sleeping. In the hospital they did all the tests, but they couldn't find any reason for the seizure. I thought the doctor must not be any good. Of course, there was a reason! Why couldn't they find it? The doctor put her on medicine, and she became a terror. She was sleepy all the time, and her personality changed from that of a lovely, affectionate little girl to that of a whiny brat. But even that was better than when the seizures came back. Her doctor tried her on many different medicines, changing them every few weeks. We were afraid to let Caroline go outside. We watched her every moment. We were frantic. We didn't know what was happening. Our child was changing before our eyes; she just wasn't Caroline any more.

"It wasn't until we worked with your medical team that we began to be more comfortable with what was going on. We learned about epilepsy and what was happening to Caroline. We began to understand seizures and their treatment, and to be less impatient with you doctors. We found ourselves becoming less overprotective, and the old Caroline began to come back. Gradually, the seizures came under control; she hasn't had one for almost four years now. Your group has taught us to be part of Caroline's team. You've taught us the importance of working with you to control her seizures. You've helped all of us deal with our fears. Caroline is doing well in school, and you've enabled us to resume a normal life.

"Parents can't cope with all these things by themselves; they need help. We needed to understand seizures, to understand the effects of the medications, but most of all we needed help to understand all the things that were happening to our child and to us. We needed your help so that we could allow our child to grow up to be as normal as possible and live with her epilepsy. We, as parents, couldn't do it ourselves. In your book, try to tell them what you told us."

We've heard this story often. Parents often come to us for a second opinion. We frequently see children who have had seizures and have been started on treatment by other physicians. What we find is that the diagnosis and medication are generally correct, but that the parents are seeking to understand. Seizures have not been fully explained. Fears and myths have not been dispelled. The future looks bleak. The most important thing we offer them is perspective. While we help the family to understand the science and psycho-social aspects of seizures, we also help them focus on the whole child, not just on the child's seizures. We want them to realize how their reactions to the seizures may be distorting family relationships. We want to help the child and the family to *live with epilepsy.*

Living with epilepsy means keeping the seizures in perspective. It means realizing that seizures are usually only a small fraction of your child's life. Living with epilepsy means avoiding handicapping your child. It means maximizing your child's assets and adjusting to the limitations, if any. Living with epilepsy may involve a struggle to find the best medication to control your child's seizures, to find optimal medical care. It may mean battling the school system or bureaucracy to get the help your child needs. It means rediscovering the joy of having a child who is learning, playing, and developing.

Over many years, we have worked as a team to develop a positive approach that incorporates both the science and the social science of seizures. This positive approach, which emphasizes what a child or adolescent *can* do rather than what he or she can't do, allows families to understand the many ramifications of epilepsy and to accept and cope with their children's seizures. This book was written to make this approach available to all families who have a child with seizures or epilepsy. Living with epilepsy will not always be easy. It will vary with your child and your child's problems. But using an optimistic approach and keeping epilepsy in perspective will make living with epilepsy better.

# Acknowledgments

This book is the product of having worked together for almost twenty years. We have learned from each other. The words and ideas no longer belong to any one individual. We have also learned from the many parents and children who have been part of our clinic as both patients and friends.

In some ways this book is part of a long tradition of comprehensive care for children with epilepsy and their families, begun at Hopkins in the 1930s under Dr. Samuel Livingston. This book's message echoes the title of one of his first books, *Living with Epilepsy.* However, our comprehensive, caring approach to epilepsy is partially due to the parents of our patients, who have helped to form our attitudes. We would like to acknowledge them as well as our own families, Jack and John Vining, Mary Pillas, and Elaine Freeman, who know how much the message of this book has meant to us and who have accepted our workaholic approach to writing it.

It is a better book because of the many friends who have read, edited and commented upon it. We give our deep gratitude to all of them for their generous contributions. They include: Drs. Peter and Carol Camfield, Ann Egerton, Nyrma Hernandez, Dr. Jody Heymann, Leigh Kingham, Ann Scherer, and Don Smith.

We are particularly indebted to Mary Edwards for her superb and tireless efforts in the preparation of multiple drafts of this manuscript, and we would also like to thank Anders Richter, editor of the Johns Hopkins University Press, for his encouragement and support, and Jeannette Hopkins, who set the manuscript free.

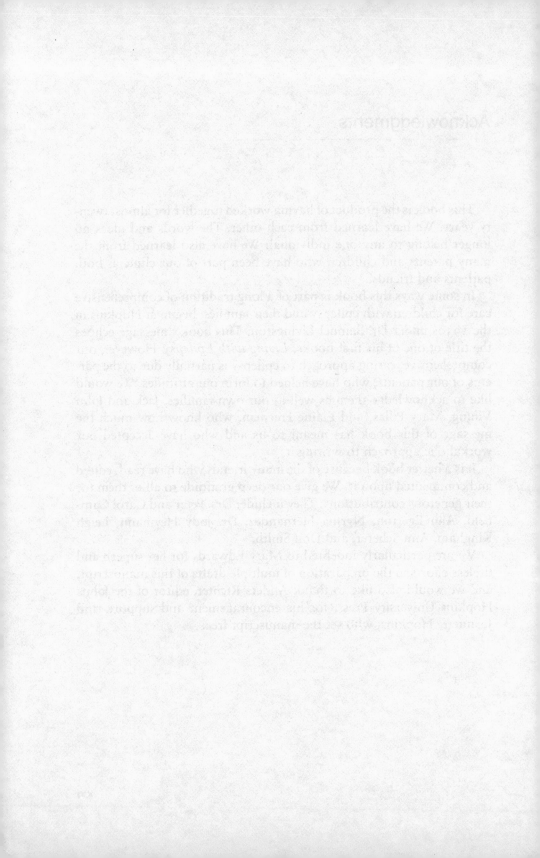

# Seizures and Epilepsy in Childhood: A Guide for Parents

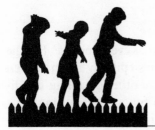

# Introduction

We see many families whose children have had a single seizure and many others whose children have epilepsy who come to us for a second opinion. There are common themes among all of these families. One theme is that the family and child are focused on the seizure or seizures; they are unable to look at the whole child and the bigger picture. Their life and their child's life has become centered primarily on the seizures. A second theme is that the families and children are overwhelmed by the mythology of epilepsy, by the fear of future handicap or retardation. Few families understand what seizures are and what they are not. They come seeking to understand what has happened and what is likely to happen.

Many physicians, even those very knowledgeable about seizures, epilepsy, and their treatment, focus on these medical aspects and do not put epilepsy in the proper perspective of the whole child and family.

We believe that no child's life should be defined by its seizures. No one is an "epileptic." The seizures and epilepsy are usually only a small portion of the child's life. We believe that to put it in perspective you must understand the brain, seizures, and how to cope with epilepsy. You must understand the mythology and how different it is from reality. Only with this understanding can you avoid handicapping your child, prevent his being handicapped by others, and allow him to reach his full potential. That is why we have written this book. While primarily for parents, it is also a book for everyone with seizures, and for all who are touched by seizures—families, teachers, and health professionals.

We hope this book will reassure you that 70 to 80 percent of children who do have epilepsy can have their seizures completely controlled

1

with medication and can function as normally as everyone else. For the smaller percentage of parents whose children's epilepsy has not been completely controlled or whose children have other disabling conditions, we hope it will help you and them to function as normally as possible to maximize their assets and minimize their disabilities.

Parents come to us with many fears: "Will my child be all right?" "Will he swallow his tongue?" "Will she die?" "Does she have a brain tumor?" "Will he be retarded?" "Can he ever lead a normal life?" "Can seizures ever be controlled?" "Can I ever leave her alone?" "Will medication make him a druggie?" All of these thoughts—and more—run through the mind of a parent whose child has had a seizure. The children themselves have similar fears: "My God! Is this going to happen again?" "What will my friends think?" "Will I ever be able to ride my bike again?" "Can I go to college?" "Can I ever drive?" "Will I be able to get married?" "What about children?"

Before we can help you to deal with these fears and put epilepsy in perspective, we must debunk the mythology. Both terms, epilepsy and seizures, carry the myths and misconceptions of centuries when people thought to be possessed by witches were confined in special colonies or shunned. They saw a child suddenly "seized," losing control, falling to the floor, his body jerking. A few minutes later this child was back to normal. What could have caused this to happen? It must have been some outside force! The devil? Not so long ago people believed this. We now know that seizures come from disruptions in the brain.

Also part of the mythology, many people still believe that epilepsy and seizures are always devastating, that they will continue to recur, that they will get worse, that the brain will be damaged, and that their child might be handicapped, become retarded, or even die. Now we know that only a small percentage of children who have a single seizure have a second seizure and, therefore, do not have epilepsy. We now know that most seizures in children can be controlled with medication, that most children outgrow their seizures and can be taken off medication. Only a minority of children with epilepsy will have difficult-to-control seizures. Most children with seizures are absolutely normal all or virtually all of the time, except during the seizure.

The mythology still persists because epilepsy remains a hidden condition. People see only the small percentage of children who are severely handicapped and who have seizures. The vast majority, whose seizures are well controlled and who function normally, do not advertise that they have epilepsy. If your neighbor's child has seizures, is on medication and is doing well, you may never even know that he has epilepsy. Only if that child has a seizure when his friends are around do they become aware of his epilepsy. His friends' parents may say, "I never knew he had epilepsy. He looks so normal!" "I thought that all children with epilepsy are retarded." "The only child I knew with seizures was in a wheelchair and never went to school." If we want to combat these old myths and prejudices, children with epilepsy and their families have to be far more comfortable and open about their disorder. Only then will the public understand that most people with epilepsy are just like themselves. Seeing only children who are disabled, you get the wrong impression. You may have no idea that most children who have epilepsy encounter no problem as a result of their seizures.

You can handicap your child if you continue to believe in the mythology. Most individuals with epilepsy *can* function normally, becoming exuberant children, vigorous adolescents, and productive adults who are free of seizures altogether. You will have to learn what protections are reasonable and realistic, and which restrictions will simply handicap your child. Avoiding overprotection will require that you understand not only seizures, but also your reaction to them, your child's reaction, and the reactions of others. You need to work actively to prevent seizures from becoming a handicap. In most cases, you can succeed.

Society's misperceptions and prejudices can handicap your child. The Epilepsy Foundation of America (EFA), the national voluntary organization for people with epilepsy, has done a wonderful job over the past decades of informing the public of the truth about epilepsy and about people with epilepsy. EFA has attempted to dispel the prejudice embodied in the term "epileptic." But prejudice can't be wholly eliminated with words and information alone. Prejudice must be fought by example as well. To overcome your prejudice truly you have to play with a child who has epilepsy, you have to go to school with him, live with him, and come to realize that he is a child, just like your own— with his own strengths, weaknesses, peculiarities, and personality. He just happens to have seizures.

The Epilepsy Foundation has tried to focus the public's attention on the children and adults whose epilepsy would otherwise be invisible. Their program emphasizes that epilepsy is usually no handicap and that children and adults who have seizures can be, and are, successful.

# Guess who's got epilepsy?

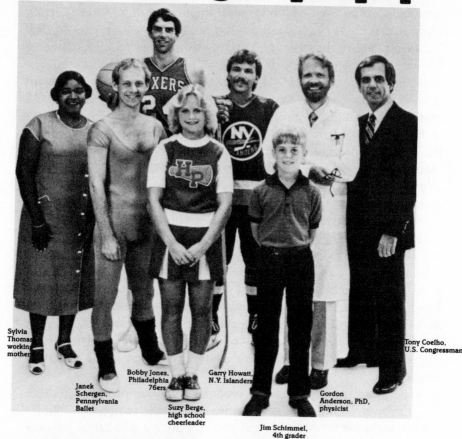

Sylvia Thomas, working mother

Janek Schergen, Pennsylvania Ballet

Bobby Jones, Philadelphia 76ers

Suzy Berge, high school cheerleader

Garry Howatt, N.Y. Islanders

Jim Schimmel, 4th grader

Gordon Anderson, PhD, physicist

Tony Coelho, U.S. Congressman

It may come as a big surprise, but all these achievers have epilepsy. Today, epilepsy isn't the handicap you might think. Thanks to medical progress, most people with epilepsy can do just about anything anybody else can do...and then some.

Get the facts. Contact your local affiliate of the Epilepsy Foundation of America.

# Epilepsy.
## It's not what you think.

Epilepsy Foundation of America, 4351 Garden City Drive, Landover, MD 20785

If your child believes in the mythology, he can handicap himself. If he allows himself to be overprotected, if he believes he can't do things because of his seizures, then he will be unable to reach his full potential. Just as you must allow him to take risks, so he must be willing to try new things. It requires self-esteem, courage, and determination to venture into the unknown, to stay at another child's house when it's possible he could have another seizure, to go to the school dance when he might be embarrassed, to apply for a job when a seizure could occur and someone might find out that he has epilepsy. Once handicapped by fear of seizures or by overprotection, it becomes difficult to break free and lead a normal life. It is far easier to prevent a handicap than to overcome it.

Helping your child to be normal will require a partnership between you and your physician. This book will help you do this. For example: your physician will do tests and may propose medication. But do not allow your physician to make all the decisions. Your doctor should be familiar with epilepsy, with the choice of medications for controlling seizures, and with their side effects. He should be willing to discuss with you the risks and benefits of each medication and of each test. Emphasize that it is your job, as the parent, to be a partner in the management—to be an informed consumer. You should ask: "Why is this test being done?" "What are its risks?" "What are the risks and benefits of treatment?" As an informed parent, you will be your child's best advocate if you understand seizures and their treatment. You must understand what epilepsy is and what it is not. You must understand what is mythology and what is fact.

We have written this book to help you understand seizures, your reaction to them, and the reaction of others. Through the stories of many of our patients we illustrate how accurate diagnosis, comprehensive treatment or management, and sensitivity to the impact of seizures can help a child and his family live better with epilepsy. With medical information you will understand the many different kinds of seizures, how the brain is organized and how it works. With knowledge of medications, you will understand your child's treatment. Only with this more complete understanding can you become a strong advocate on the team that is helping your child.

# Part One

# Why Do Seizures and Epilepsy Occur?

# 1. How the Brain Works:
## Understanding Seizures and Why There Are So Many Types

For most people the brain is a black box, a mystifying organ sitting between the ears. For most people seizures are sudden, frightening events that come from this black box like "static" on a radio or a lightning bolt of electricity. When the brain and its dysfunctions are thought of in this fashion, all you as a parent or a patient can do is mechanically to give or take the medication that your doctor prescribes and hope that it is the right thing to do and that it will stop these terrible events.

We believe that parents and children should be participants in their own care. We believe that both the brain and epilepsy are understandable and that when you understand, you can be a far more effective and helpful participant.

Before you can understand epilepsy and participate in your child's care or your own care, you have to understand how the brain works and how and why the disruptions of its function, called seizures, occur.

### Society: A Model for Disruptions and Seizures

The brain is a society of cells called "neurons"; it works through the interactions of individual neurons, one with the other. Brief disruptions in the brain, that is, seizures, alter the interactions of these cells. To understand normal brain function and the disturbances of function called seizures, it may be helpful to consider another complex but more familiar structure—society, with its interactions and disruptions.

We all live in "society" and also in smaller communities: a family, a neighborhood, a church, a workplace, a town, a country. We are each members of multiple communities. Each of us is different: male or female, black or white, young or old. Our interactions create the social environment. So, too, is the brain a society, one composed of millions of individual cells (neurons), each with its own characteristics, each with its own interactions, each influencing and being influenced by its neighbors and by its local community. The brain has many different regions or communities, and within these regions cells relate to each other in different ways. The regions also influence one another.

Throughout most brains, as within most societies, these interactions occur in an orderly fashion, with few disruptions. But, occasionally, in a society, there are disruptions like a holiday, a parade, an accident, a fire, a strike. Some interruptions occur more often in some communities than in others; unpleasant disruptions, for example, occur more frequently in big cities with a greater diversity of people and more multiple interactions than in rural environments. After these "blips" in the normal pattern of life, communities usually resume their previous tempos quickly and return to normal activities.

But occasionally disruptions are more intense. Perhaps lives are lost in a fire. The community is disrupted, its ordinary functions come to a halt, it grieves, it holds memorial services. Interactions among citizens are changed, not forever probably, but for a longer period of time than if a parade has passed by. The response of the community will depend on multiple factors—its ethnic heritage, its size, its age, and the interrelationships within the community. Some disruptions spread more widely and involve larger segments of the community, the region, the country, or the entire society. A strike of bus drivers or rail workers may affect the whole region. A march for a popular cause may mobilize a community and a nation.

Similarly, within the brain, communities of cells and areas of the brain interact at their own pace—different paces for different regions. These interactions in the brain are assessed by the EEG (electroencephalogram), a record of the minute amounts of electrical activity that brain cells give off as they relate to each other. The normal EEG appears as a series of wiggly lines, with rhythms seeming to move almost at random across the paper. The electrical activity measured varies from one area of the brain to another. But on rare occasions a "blip" appears among these wiggly lines, a small jolt of electricity, a "spike." This spike is like the minor episode, such as an automobile accident, that disrupts a community briefly. The brain quickly resumes its activity. Such spikes on the EEG are of little consequence. Only when they recur frequently in one area of the brain is it evident that that particular community of cells is prone to disruption.

When an electrical disturbance involves one area of the brain it may be visible in twitches of the hand. It may spread throughout one side of the brain, a unilateral seizure, or it may spread throughout the whole brain, causing a generalized seizure. Each of these disturbances is a single seizure, but a single seizure is not epilepsy. Two or more seizures are called epilepsy.

Within society there are soapbox orators or fiery speakers who stand on street corners, trying to cause disturbances, urging people to "take action." Most people walk by. Occasionally, some people stop, listen, and then walk on. Some of the audience may get excited, but action virtually never ensues; they don't change their behavior and a demonstration does not begin. But on rare occasions, this fiery speaker arouses the surrounding crowd and a march or a demonstration occurs. It will not happen solely because he is an inspired speaker, but because of the interaction between the speaker and the audience. The interaction must be sufficient to rouse the crowd to action. In the brain tiny scars, or small abnormalities, are like the fiery speakers in a crowd. Usually this abnormal tissue causes no disruptions or change in brain function. Just as a crowd may pay no attention to a speaker, so the surrounding cells may fail to respond to the abnormality, and then nothing happens. Change in function, a seizure, requires the interaction of the abnormal area *and* the community.

This susceptibility of surrounding neurons is termed "threshold." To understand a spike or a seizure, we must understand the level of arousal or "threshold" of the surrounding cells. If the brain's threshold is lowered it is more susceptible to the effects of the "fiery speaker," the scar, and a seizure is more likely to occur in the community of the brain. If the electrical activity from a scar interacts with mildly aroused surrounding cells, a local disturbance may appear as recurrent spikes on the EEG, but this is not a seizure. A seizure is a paroxysmal electrical discharge of neurons in the brain *resulting in alteration of function or behavior.*

The alteration of function or behavior that occurs in a seizure will depend on the magnitude and type of the disruption or disorganization and on the "community" of the brain in which it occurs. Local disruptions of brain function are called "partial" seizures because only part of the brain is involved. Since each area of the brain has a different function, the manifestations of an electrical disruption or seizure will differ, depending on which area of the brain is involved. When a partial seizure affects one area of the brain, the manifestations may be twitching of the thumb, hand, or face. If it affects another, there may be a tingling sensation, a peculiar smell, an unusual taste. In other areas, the seizure may lead to changes in behavior—staring or alterations of awareness. All such seizures are caused by local (contained) disruption of normal electrical activity.

But, as in a society, so a seizure or demonstration may not remain confined to a local region. Depending on its intensity and on the threshold of the brain, the disturbance or seizure may become sufficiently severe to involve a large part of the brain or, indeed, the whole brain and become a generalized seizure.

Just as we do not understand exactly why demonstrations begin, spread, and end in a society, we also do not yet completely understand the factors that maintain the seizure focus in the brain or the interactions with the "crowd" of surrounding neurons. How does excitement, lack of sleep, or a fever alter the threshold of the surrounding cells? What genetic and environmental factors influence the "threshold"? If we understood the multiple factors and interactions that cause disruptions in the brain, and the factors that cause these disruptions to stop, we could probably prevent seizures from occurring altogether. But we do not.

## Why Do Seizures Occur?

Only by understanding something about the physiology of the brain—how it works—and its anatomy can we understand the many different types of seizures that can occur and consider why they happen.

The brain works on electricity, with neurons (nerve cells) communicating and interacting by discharging or "firing" tiny electrical impulses along interconnecting "wires" called axons. The electrical impulse results in the release of a chemical called a neurotransmitter from the axon's ending or terminal (Fig. 1.1) that then interacts with the next cell. These chemicals (neurotransmitters) can be excitatory, that is make the next cell more likely to fire (Fig. 1.2A) or inhibitory, that is

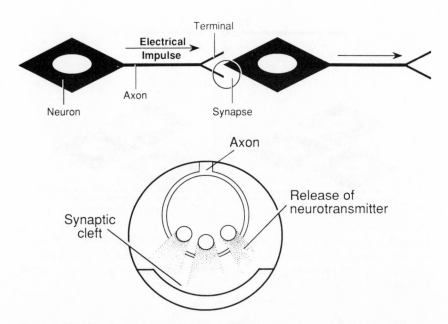

**Figure 1.1.** Communication between nerve cells. Neurons or nerve cells communicate by discharging electrical impulses along interconnecting axons, resulting in the release of a neurotransmitter, which floats across the space between cells (the synaptic cleft) and activates the next cell.

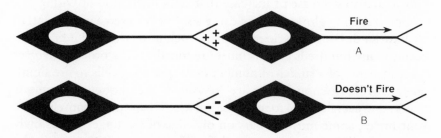

**Figure 1.2.** Excitation (A) and inhibition (B) of neuron. Some neurotransmitters, released by electrical impulse of neurons, may excite the next cell and cause it to fire (A); others inhibit the next cell and make it less likely to fire (B). The total of the excitatory (+) and inhibitory (−) impulses that influence each cell determines whether the cell will be stimulated to fire (its threshold). When the excitatory (+) impulses outnumber the inhibitory (−) impulses, the cell will fire.

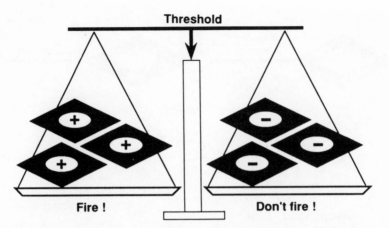

**Figure 1.3.** Threshold. The balance between exciting (+) and inhibitory (−) influences. A loss of inhibitory influences or increase in excitatory influences may cause a cell to fire. Similarly, a loss of exciting influences or an increase in inhibition may cause a cell not to fire.

cause the next cell to be less likely to fire (Fig. 1.2B). Each cell has many thousands of endings; some of them (excitatory) are telling the cell to say "yes" and increasing the chance of that cell's "firing." There are some endings on the cell that say "no" (inhibitory), decreasing the chance of that cell's "firing". The balance of these excitatory and inhibitory impulses influences its threshold, or how readily that cell can be stimulated to fire (Fig. 1.3). The increase or loss of influences saying "no" can also decrease or increase that cell's likelihood of "firing."

One cell firing alone does not cause a seizure or even a movement, as we have said. For a muscle movement, such as a twitch of a finger, to occur, many hundreds of cells must fire together. The process involves "recruitment" of a sufficient number of neighboring cells to fire simultaneously. If not enough cells are "recruited" then not enough muscle fibers contract (shorten) to move the muscle. When you purposely move your finger, some muscle fibers on one side of the finger joint slowly contract (pull) in a coordinated fashion. The movement is controlled by the relaxation of muscle fibers on the other side of the joint (fired by different brain cells). This coordination and interaction of different groups of brain cells that control the muscle fibers on each side of the finger joint allow you to manipulate finger movement. If, however, one group of cells in the brain fires without the controlling influence of other cells your finger jerks or twitches. This is what happens in some types of seizures (Fig. 1.4).

The brain functions normally when there is interaction of many cells. When a sufficient number of cells work together, an "event" occurs. What the event will be is determined by which cells are firing. If the firing cells are in the motor area of the brain, the event may be the movement of a finger, hand, or foot; if it is in the sensory area, it may be a feeling like a tingle or a burning. In other areas it may be a taste, or a

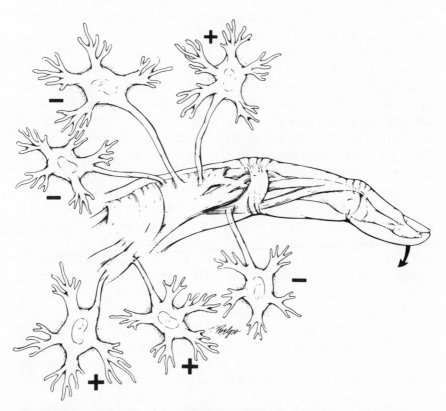

**Figure 1.4.** Muscle twitches and movements. Movement of a finger requires coordination of cells in the brain to achieve smooth coordination of muscles on both sides of a joint. Drawing shows a smooth downward movement of the finger because the contraction of the muscles on the underside, stimulated by nerve cells firing (+), is accompanied by relaxation of muscles on top of the finger, caused by nerve cells inhibited from firing (−). In a seizure, all cells on the underside might fire suddenly, causing the finger to jerk rather than to move smoothly downward.

smell, or a memory. These normal human experiences occur when specialized parts of the brain are sufficiently excited.

A seizure occurs when the balance between excitation and inhibition is lost. A motor seizure, for example, happens when a sufficient number of cells spontaneously fire together and produce a sudden movement, a jerk. Not all sudden movements are seizures. A seizure is usually the result of repetitive firing of these same cells; when in the motor area repetitive firing leads to the rhythmic, repetitive jerking of a group of muscles.

Other types of seizures occur when cells from other areas of the brain fire simultaneously. The type of seizure depends on how many cells fire and which area of the brain is affected.

The truth is that we don't really know *why* a seizure occurs. We understand much about how the brain works and what a seizure is, how it happens, but not always why. We can explain how single cells fire, how they communicate with other cells, and a lot about the chemical and electrical makeup of neurons. We know that a cell's function is affected by its chemical environment. We know, for example, that oxygen and glucose (sugar) are required to keep neurons healthy and working; with insufficient oxygen or glucose cells may fire abnormally and cause a seizure. Lack of blood supply to a part of the brain, such as after a stroke, can cause seizures by reducing the oxygen and chemicals necessary to keep these nerve cells functioning normally. Significant changes in important body chemicals such as calcium and magnesium can cause seizures; so can a lack of certain vitamins. These chemical changes may provoke a disturbance in the brain, or a single seizure, by influencing the threshold for firing, but they rarely cause epilepsy.

A high fever, a blow to the head, or an infection of the brain such as meningitis or encephalitis, can provoke an isolated seizure by causing sufficient disruption of surrounding cells. But most seizures are the result of the *interaction* between the fiery speaker and the crowd, between the provocation to the brain and the surrounding neurons.

## The Importance of Threshold

The threshold is the level of excitement at which a neuron will fire. As we have indicated, a cell's threshold is determined by the excitatory and inhibitory influences upon it. The seizure threshold is the level at which

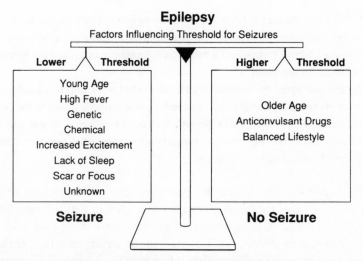

**Figure 1.5.** Factors influencing threshold for seizures. While genetic factors may be most important, factors such as age and fever may lower the threshold, making a child more likely to have a seizure. Factors such as older age and anticonvulsants may decrease the chances of a seizure.

the brain will have a seizure, at which multiple cells will fire simultaneously (Fig. 1.5).

Chemical factors, lack of oxygen, low calcium can lower the threshold as can fever, excitement, lack of sleep. In general, the brain has a large margin of safety to protect it from misfiring. The size of this margin of safety is determined genetically. As a consequence, some people are closer to the threshold than others. In individuals with a previously low genetic threshold, fever may cause an event known as a "febrile," or fever-induced, seizure. Seizures can be produced in anyone if the temperature becomes sufficiently high (107° to 108°F) and if the brain becomes sufficiently excited. In those with a lower genetic resistance or threshold, a febrile seizure may occur at a temperature of 103° or 104°. If the threshold of an individual is quite low, a seizure may occur with only slightly increased excitement, at 101° or 102°. Similarly, mild head trauma may cause a seizure in a child with a low genetic threshold, whereas it would take far more severe head trauma to cause a seizure in a child with a higher threshold.

❏ **Mrs. Circiello was driving the children to school when a truck hit the car broadside. Both children in the back seat hit their heads against the side of the car. Johnny's friend Roger had a tonic-clonic seizure. Johnny was fine except for the bump on his head.**

**Why did one child have a seizure and the other not? One possibility is that Roger hit his head harder and this caused a greater disturbance in the brain. A second possibility is that, since Roger's father has seizures, Roger has inherited a lower threshold. Therefore, although his injury was the same as Johnny's, it was sufficient to trigger a seizure.**

The threshold for a seizure is dependent also on age. Young children have lower seizure thresholds than adults. That is why young children are more likely to have a seizure when they get a fever and why most epilepsy begins in childhood. The increase in threshold with age may be the reason why most epilepsy that has begun in childhood is outgrown.

Emotional factors and other physical factors also influence a child's margin of safety. Excitement in response to a birthday party or a trip, or agitation caused by an argument or punishment, or anxiety during an exam may lower the individual's margin of safety and cause a seizure. So may lack of sleep in an individual whose threshold is already low. Such interactions of genetic threshold and environmental influences may explain many single, presumably "spontaneous," seizures.

Chemical changes in the blood, such as low blood sugar or low calcium levels, make neurons more susceptible to firing but are usually insufficient of themselves to produce seizures except in a "low-threshold, seizure-prone" child.

Although the margin of safety is largely determined by a child's genetic makeup, it varies from time to time and day to day depending on factors like the above. Whatever the margin of safety is at a given point in time, the threshold may be exceeded and a seizure result if there is an additional inciting influence such as head trauma. Thus, a greater injury, a lower margin of safety, or a combination of the two may result in a seizure at a specific time. *Anyone can have a seizure if the trauma or disturbance is sufficiently great to exceed his threshold.*

On the other side of the scale (Fig. 1.5), anticonvulsant drugs, for example, increase the margin of safety and decrease the chance of a seizure's occurring. If medication is accidentally forgotten, then the margin of safety decreases, the child is closer to his threshold, and a seizure becomes more likely.

Thus, multiple interacting factors influence the susceptibility to seizures in any individual child, and their interactions may play a role in determining why seizures occur and recur at a specific time. As we learn more about the brain and its mechanisms of control we will understand more about threshold and about an individual's margin of safety. If we could increase that margin of safety, or increase the threshold, then we could better prevent seizures.

These are many of the aspects of WHY a seizure, a disruption in the brain, occurs, but where in the brain it occurs and how it spreads are equally important because they determine the type of seizures.

# Part Two
# Diagnosing and Treating Seizures

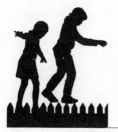

# 2. How We Diagnose a Seizure and Decide What It Will Mean for Your Child

A seizure, as we have seen, is a sudden alteration in behavior or in motor function caused by an electrical discharge from the brain.

It should be very easy to diagnose a seizure since it is simply a sudden change in behavior or motor function. But sometimes it's not that simple; people have sudden changes in behavior all the time. Sometimes children faint, daydream, or fall down. How do you tell if those events were seizures? *The only way to diagnose a seizure is to take a very careful history of the event that has occurred.*

That's why doctors ask all those questions. What was the child doing when it happened? What was the first thing that was noticed? What happened next? What was the child doing during the episode? The doctor may ask you to demonstrate what you saw (if you saw it). Was the child trembling, making rapid movements of the arms or legs, or were the child's arms or legs jerking rhythmically? What was the child like afterward? Was she tired? Was there a headache? Did the child wet herself during the spell? While none of these findings is specific for a seizure, the pattern may make the physician more or less suspicious that the episode was a seizure.

*There is no diagnostic test for a seizure or for epilepsy. The diagnosis rests solely on the physician's interpretation of the history of the episode which occurred.*

Since physicians rarely have the opportunity to see the seizure events for themselves, they must depend on the observation of parents or other witnesses to the episode. Most of these observers have never seen a true seizure and are upset and panicked by what they have seen. When they relay the information through third parties, the story can grow more lurid or lose important details. Frequently events occur at school or when the child is with friends. The person who actually saw the "seizure" will give more useful responses if he or she is calmly questioned about exactly what happened to your child. This is one of the reasons why you are such an important member of the team. The physician can't make a diagnosis without good information. You may need to talk to teachers, friends, or even other children who saw what happened.

Let us give you an example of how difficult it may be to determine whether a particular episode was a seizure and how we think about the episode's importance for the child's future.

❑ **Jane is thirteen years old, and the nurse is cleaning her arm with alcohol in preparation for taking the blood tests ordered by her physician. The nurse takes out the syringe and needle and Jane says, "Wait a minute, I don't feel well." She looks pale and sweaty, then collapses in the chair. She stiffens and has jerking of her arms and legs that lasts perhaps a minute. Was that a seizure? "Yes," the physician says. "That is what is called 'convulsive syncope.' Jane fainted, just as many people faint when blood is taken. In some people, fainting is enough to trigger a brief seizure. It's nothing to worry about. She'll be fine."**

That diagnosis was easy. Jane's seizure occurred because of fainting. The episode was witnessed from the start by people trained to observe carefully. They heard Jane say she didn't feel well. They saw her become pale and sweaty *before* losing consciousness. It was clear to them that Jane fainted and then had a seizure. The episode occurred in a situation where fainting is not uncommon. But suppose Jane had been sitting in the hot sun with her friends at a baseball game when the episode occurred? Could she have been drinking beer or taking drugs? Would her friends have noted the paleness and sweating before she fainted, became stiff, and had the brief jerking movements? If they hadn't noticed the fainting and had only seen the jerking, your doctor might not have known why the seizure occurred and would have been concerned that it might recur. He could not have been as confident in saying that it was convulsive syncope.

## Was It a Seizure?

After a careful, detailed history, the physician should be able to say one of three things:

   1. "That episode was clearly a seizure."

OR

   2. "That was clearly not a seizure. It sounds to me like a fainting spell (breathholding spell, etc)."

OR

   3. "I'm not sure what that episode was. I don't think it was a seizure, but let's wait and see if it recurs. If it does recur, I want you to observe him carefully and look for . . . "

Even if a single episode was a seizure, it may not be important for your child's future since most single seizures do not recur or require treatment. If episodes are recurring, it should not take long for careful observation to determine their true nature. If infrequent and not interfering with the child's life, they are less important. Rare episodes will either disappear as mysteriously as they appeared, or they will become sufficiently obvious and frequent to allow proper diagnosis.

*Many people have been told they have seizures and, subsequently, have been treated with medication because of incorrect interpretation of single events, such as fainting. When in doubt about an event or about the circumstances of it, it is usually better to wait to see if a similar event recurs. It is better to live with uncertainty than to allow yourself or your physician to be too eager to label the event and begin your treatment. If there is doubt about the nature of the event or events, whether or not your child is on medication, you should explore this further with your doctor. Even when your child clearly has had a seizure, different seizures will have different meanings for the child's future. The meaning may well depend on the context in which the seizure occurred. He may not need extensive evaluation and medication. Decisions about these may depend on the circumstances in which the seizure or seizures occurred.*

## Provoked and Unprovoked Seizures

❏ **Your child is playing outside when his friend comes banging at the door. "Come quick!" the friend shouts. "Something's happened to Bobby!" You run** and find Bobby on the edge of the playground jerking his arms and legs and making gurgling sounds. "Was that a seizure?" you ask your physician later. "It certainly sounds like one," she replies. "We have to be concerned that Bobby might have another one. If he does, then he has epilepsy—by definition." If after talking to Bobby's friend she learns that Bobby was climbing a tree, fell, and hit his head, she might answer differently. "I think Bobby had a slight concussion and a brief seizure, what we call a 'post-traumatic seizure.' These brief seizures after a child hits his head are not uncommon and rarely recur. I think that this is what we call a provoked seizure. I don't believe he has epilepsy or will have epilepsy."

It is not the mere occurrence of a seizure but also the *circumstances* under which the seizure occurs that determine if a child is likely to have more seizures. Furthermore, the child must have two or more seizures or he has not got epilepsy.

If a child has several seizures during an episode of meningitis, or after a head injury, or with diarrhea and dehydration, or with other acute "illnesses," these seizures are termed "provoked" seizures or "symptomatic" seizures, ones that have a defined cause, just as Jane's seizure after fainting was a "provoked" seizure. The acute brain disturbance that caused them will disappear or be cured and the seizures should not recur.

Although acute conditions such as a head injury or meningitis *can* cause permanent damage to the brain, and that damage *can* later lead to "unprovoked" recurrent seizures—i.e., epilepsy—permanent damage followed later by epilepsy is not a consequence of acute "symptomatic" seizures in children.

## Episodes Often Mistaken for Seizures

Many changes in motor function or behavior are commonly mistaken for seizures. These include fainting, tics, and other sudden jerking movements, breathholding spells, migraine headaches, and episodic changes in behavior. Doctors who are aware of these types of behaviors can take a careful history and can usually separate them from seizures.

## Is It Fainting or a Seizure?

❏ It had been a long church service and, as usual, Rebecca had almost been late. Her alarm had not gone off, and when her mother had called her there had barely been time to get dressed. No time for breakfast. Her mother told me, "The sermon was long and dull, and she remembers standing for the hymns and feeling dizzy. The next thing she remembers is waking up outside the church. She doesn't remember passing out. The paramedic who happened to be there asked me if Rebecca had epilepsy. Does she? You'll tell me the truth, Doctor, won't you?"

Fainting spells are commonly misdiagnosed as seizures. Indeed, some people have been treated for "epilepsy" for years when they had simply fainted. Fainting is caused by lack of blood going to the brain. Since one of the brain's important activities is to maintain consciousness and posture, when there is not enough blood the person may become dizzy and slump to the floor. This decrease of bloodflow to the brain may be due to slowing of, or even brief pauses in, the heart rate. Or it may result from prolonged standing, with the blood becoming pooled in the legs or in the abdomen with not enough blood available to pump to the brain. Or it could result from anemia, with insufficient red blood cells to carry oxygen to the brain.

In each case, the lack of blood initially causes a paleness, followed by sweating. The person feels "lightheaded," or dizzy. The room seems to spin, and he or she slumps (not crashes) to the ground. As soon as the person is lying down, the heart does not have to pump blood up to the head, the blood supply to the brain is immediately increased, and within seconds he regains consciousness. He will usually still be pale and sweaty, may briefly be confused, and may still feel weak. Even though he has had a change in motor function and consciousness, he has not, however, had a seizure since that change was not caused by abnormal electrical activity in the brain.

Fainting can precede and cause a seizure, as in Jane's case, or occur without a seizure, as we have seen in Rebecca's story. Fainting spells may occur when someone hasn't eaten, when someone gives blood, or occasionally after insufficient sleep or after extreme tension or anxiety or with overventilation due to anxiety. Fainting spells can occur in individuals who have low blood pressure who stand up too fast.

When we understand the circumstances and the sequence of events, we should be able to distinguish easily between convulsive syncope (seizures with fainting) and other seizures. The preceding paleness and sweatiness described are typical of fainting but not of seizures. Wetting oneself is more common during seizures than after fainting, but can occur in both situations. On the other hand, any person who bites his tongue may be having a seizure since someone who faints does not bite his tongue.

*When the sequence of events is unclear, the physician will probably want to wait before making a diagnosis since it is better to be uncertain than to label the event "a seizure."* If the child continues to have these episodes, either the nature of the spells will become clear or further tests are indicated to determine the appropriate diagnosis and treatment. An EEG *does not* differentiate between fainting and seizures unless an episode occurs when the EEG is running.

Fainting spells are not considered seizures unless they are accompanied by stiffening or jerking. If they are accompanied by stiffening or jerking, they are considered provoked seizures but are not considered serious since they are unlikely to recur except in similar circumstances. They are not considered epilepsy and do not respond to medications used to treat epilepsy. This "convulsive syncope" or convulsive fainting has no more meaning than the fainting episode itself.

## Is It Daydreaming or a Seizure?

❑ **"Phillip has become forgetful," you tell your doctor. "The other day we were cleaning up the yard, and I asked him to pick up a pile of leaves. He just went on raking up the leaves. I shouted at him a second time, but he ignored me. I got mad, but when I went over to him he claimed he hadn't even heard me. He seems to be doing that a lot lately."**

**"It could be a lot of things," your physician replies. "As you know, adolescents often have selective hearing. It could be that he was listening to his Walkman, or daydreaming, or just tired of being nagged. Could he be taking drugs? Since you say that he has been having a lot of these things, I suppose that they could be seizures, the kind we call absence or petit mal. Let me get him to overbreathe (hyperventilate) a little bit and see if we can produce a spell."**

A teacher may describe a child as "daydreaming a lot" or as "not paying attention." Or, on occasion, a child herself may report that she is missing short segments of her lessons or brief parts of a TV program. Without seeing a staring spell, it will be difficult to interpret such brief events. Such spells may often be precipitated by hyperventilation in the physician's office; if an episode can be made to occur, the physician can see the spell and interpret for herself.

Daydreaming can be very difficult to differentiate from the brief lapses in attention caused by absence seizures. We will discuss this further in Chapter 6. Daydreaming, however, is common in situations which are boring or when a child is tired; absence seizures can occur at any time. Absence seizures may be seen at meal times and interrupt a conversation or eating, whereas in these situations a child is unlikely to daydream. Daydreaming can usually be interrupted by calling the child's name or touching the child. Absence seizures cannot be interrupted.

## Tics

❏ "Joshua started these funny movements a couple of weeks ago, Doctor. It's just in his face. He sort of makes these funny faces, not all the time, but they're getting more frequent. I've yelled at him to stop. They drive me crazy. He'll stop for a little while and then do it again. Now he's started jerking his shoulder and grunting. Do you think he's getting epilepsy?"

Tics, like seizures, are sudden, paroxysmal movements. They are usually quicker movements than seizures themselves. While they most commonly affect the head and face, they may affect other parts of the body as well. Unlike seizures, they can be voluntarily controlled for periods of time. A tic may be simple, so that the movement looks like a twitch of a muscle or group of muscles, or it may be a complex pattern of movements. Unlike seizures, the recurrent movements are stereotyped. Seizures rarely look exactly the same from episode to episode because of the variations in spread of the electrical activity in the brain. But most tics are reproduced exactly and should, therefore, be easy to identify. Medications can be used to treat severe tics, but they are different from those used to treat seizures.

## Myoclonic Jerks

❏ "We were lying down together on the couch, watching TV, and Carl was just dozing off, when suddenly he had this big jerk, like a seizure. His arms and legs went out like he was struck by a jolt of electricity. Then he was awake, and just like nothing had happened. This is the third one of these I've seen in the past few months. This isn't epilepsy, is it? I'm worried because Carl's uncle has epilepsy."

Myoclonic jerks are sudden movements, usually of an arm, leg, or both arms or legs, often occurring just as an individual is falling asleep. These are called "sleep myoclonus," and they are common and normal. Myoclonic jerks during waking hours are less common, but unless frequent they should be of little concern. Frequent myoclonic jerks can be a form of epilepsy (see Chapter 6).

### Breathholding Spells

❏ "Sarah used to be such a good baby, but now she's got 'the terrible two's.' First, she started with temper tantrums, crying when she didn't get her way. Then she began to hold her breath and turn bluish, and I'd just pick her up and she would settle down. But now something different is happening, and I'm scared. Yesterday she was running and tripped and bumped her head. She started to cry, then she just held her breath and couldn't breathe. She turned blue, then she became stiff and arched her back and started to jerk all over. I'm sure she had a seizure."

Have you ever noticed that when your child cries hard she will often exhale and seem to hold her breath for a long time before taking another breath? This is normal, even when the delay before the next breath seems interminable. For reasons that are unclear, some children hold their breath longer than others and turn blue or stiffen their bodies and arch their backs or even lose consciousness. This is a "breathholding spell." In a few children, at the end of the breathholding, a seizure may occur with stiffening and jerking.

The blood has lost some of its oxygen while the child is holding her breath, and that is why she turns blue. With insufficient oxygen, a child loses consciousness. If the lack of oxygen is severe or if the child's seizure threshold is low, a seizure may be provoked.

A breathholding spell is virtually always caused by minor trauma, like a fall or bump, or by frustration when, for example, a toy is taken away or the child is punished. In such cases, stiffening and jerking are always preceded by crying and by breathholding. Seizures of epilepsy, on the other hand, are *never* brought on by such trauma or frustration and are *never* preceded by similar crying. Breathholding episodes, even when accompanied by seizures, do not need to be treated with anticonvulsant medicine, and do not respond to such medication. Typical breathholding spells do not require any laboratory examination. Treatment of breathholding spells consists of careful explanation of their benign nature, with reassurance that the child will not die, does not need resuscitation, and will outgrow the spells.

When the oxygen level drops, the child automatically starts breathing again on her own and the brain is protected. While very frightening to the parent, breathholding episodes will NOT result in brain damage.

Sometimes these breathholding spells can be aborted or prevented by diverting the child's attention. Also, since the crying and frustration that cause these spells are reinforced by parental overprotection in fear that a spell will reoccur, behavioral modification should be taught to the family by the physician or by a behavioral psychologist. Parents should learn to ignore the crying and reward the child's good behavior, and not reward the tantrum and breathholding with attention and concern. The spells will probably then decrease in frequency and the child will outgrow them without long-term consequences as the central nervous system matures.

There is a second form of these spells that is misnamed "pallid breathholding spells," usually occurring after trauma such as a bump on the head. The child suddenly stops what he has been doing, turns pale, and may fall down. Occasionally the child will then arch his back and rarely experience jerking movements. Such spells are not preceded by crying, breathholding, or turning blue. They are caused by "vasovagal syncope," that is, fainting because of overactivity of the normal reflex that slows the heart rate. If the heart beat slows sufficiently, not enough blood is pumped to the brain and the child loses consciousness and stiffens. These "pallid breathholding spells" are the infancy and childhood counterpart of fainting when blood is drawn. The slowing of the heart rate can often be reproduced in the physician's office by pressing on the child's closed eye. If a child has an overactive vagal nerve reflex, the physician will hear a dramatic slowing of the heart rate, at times even a brief pause between heart beats. If an EKG (electrocardiogram) is running at the time, the increasingly longer interval between heart beats can be documented.

Although they are frightening, pallid spells are usually benign and will be outgrown. Only rarely, when the spells are quite frequent, is it necessary to consider treatment, but not with anticonvulsants since these spells are not seizures. The appropriate medications are those that block the action of the vagus nerve and prevent the slowing of the heart.

## Migraine Headaches

❑ "Lisa has been having headaches for a year or more, Doctor, but these past few months they've become more frequent. Now she has one several times a week, and she is missing a lot of school. She says that they are all over her head, but mainly start behind her eyes. She has to come home from school and feels sick to her stomach. She usually goes to bed and wants the lights off because they bother her eyes. Sometimes she will throw up, and then she feels better. She sleeps for a few hours and then is fine. She hasn't had any seizures for almost two years now, but the headache is like the ones she sometimes had after her big seizures. Do you think she could have migraine? I used to have migraine attacks when I was young."

Migraine headaches are not uncommon in children but often do not resemble adult migraine. They rarely are unilateral or associated with warnings (auras) such as flashing lights or unilateral sensory symptoms. Migraine headaches in children may build up as pounding headaches, with nausea, and sometimes with vomiting. The child usually tries to avoid light, goes to his room, lies down, and goes to sleep. Such headaches typically last for hours. In children these headaches are often bilateral. This kind of an attack is not like a seizure, but the episode is sometimes confused with a seizure when the headache component is less severe or when nausea and vomiting are less prominent.

Migraine commonly occurs in families, hence there appears to be a genetic predisposition. Longer duration of the episode and nausea suggest migraine. The presence of other seizures may indicate, however, that the headaches are related to a seizure. Both the headache of the migraine attack and the headache after a seizure can be similar since both are caused by dilation of blood vessels in the brain.

The EEG may be abnormal both in persons with migraine and in those with seizures; therefore, the EEG is an unreliable procedure for deciding which kind of episode has occurred. In some instances, it may not be possible at all to differentiate between migraine headaches and headaches related to seizures (epileptic cephalgia). Indeed, as noted, migraine and seizures may coexist. Migraine is more common in those individuals and families with a history of seizures, and seizures are more common in those with a history of migraine. If the doctor thinks these events are more likely to be seizures, he may suggest a trial of anticonvulsant medication; a good response to these drugs suggests that the events were, indeed, seizures. If the doctor thinks these are more likely migraine attacks, he will prescribe antimigraine drugs. Again, a good response to this medication will suggest that he was right. Migraine has been known to respond to some anticonvulsants, but it is doubtful that seizures will respond to some medications now used to treat migraine.

## Paroxysmal Behavioral Disturbances

☐ "Peter has been a terror for years now. We've had him to several psychologists, and we're on our third psychiatrist. Now he's in a residential school for further evaluation. Something has to be done to control these outbursts before he kills someone. They did an EEG, and now they say that this is epilepsy because the EEG is abnormal. I've read about epilepsy, and Peter has never had a seizure. It's just that when someone frustrates him, or does something he doesn't like, he erupts like a volcano. There's no controlling him. He hits and bites and punches. I'm afraid he'll hurt somebody. Gradually he'll calm down and act as if he's sorry. Could this be epilepsy? I almost hope so, since then we'll have medicine to treat him."

Sudden outbursts of bizarre, often violent behavior are not uncommon among emotionally disturbed children and also among those who are mildly or moderately retarded. Psychiatrists often ask their neurological colleagues if such episodes can be seizures. *The answer is virtually always no!* Studies have shown that apparently intentional violence almost never occurs during a seizure. If, during the confusion that commonly occurs during the "post-ictal" state, that is, after the seizure, a child is restrained or threatened, a child may react in a combative but random fashion. In this post-ictal, confused state, the child does not mean to fight back or even understand what he is doing.

Episodic behavioral outbursts are almost always precipitated by an event or by frustration. Seizures never are. Seizures usually have a post-ictal state in which the child is tired or confused. Behavioral outbursts never do. However, the EEG obtained between seizures or behavioral episodes may be either normal or abnormal and, therefore, does not help differentiate seizures from behavioral outbursts. Spikes on an EEG (see Chapter 7) can be observed in children who never have seizures.

*Repeated episodic behavioral changes, in the absence of obvious seizures, are virtually never seizures and, therefore, do not respond to anticonvulsants.*

Rare patients have confused even the best neurologists. In these cases, trying to capture the episode on video-EEG monitoring may be the only method of ascertaining what is a seizure and what is not. Needless to say, the same individual may experience behavioral problems and seizures also.

## Pseudo-seizures

Psychological symptoms may cause intentional or subconscious episodic alterations in function or in consciousness that are mistaken for seizures but are *not,* in fact, of electrical origin and hence are not seizures. Although they may closely imitate seizures, such nonelectrical episodes are "pseudo-seizures."

❏ **"I'm glad we finally got an appointment with you. Leslie's schoolwork is deteriorating, and the medications do not seem to be helping her seizures. Ever since our divorce she has had seizures, and her doctors have tried every combination of medication. Nothing has helped. Every time she spends a weekend at her father's house she has a seizure. She falls to the ground, flails her legs and arms, and doesn't respond when we shout at her. I know that her EEG is abnormal. Isn't there something you can do to help? Is she a candidate for surgery?"**

Does Leslie really have seizures? It's hard to be sure. Her doctor might ask for a more precise description of the "flailing." He would want to check to see what abnormalities, if any, appear on the EEG. He would be suspicious that the episodes occurred only at her father's house and began after the divorce.

As with seizures, pseudo-seizures require therapy, but therapy that is quite different from that used for "true" seizures. Our first approach would be to take a much more careful history of the events that occurred and the circumstances under which they occurred. We would also take a separate history from Leslie. "Were you taking your medicine at your father's house? Do special things cause these episodes, for example an argument or a fight?" Depending on our sense of this story, we would try to decide whether these were real or pseudo-seizures.

Since Leslie is having problems in school, and since the medications for presumed seizures have been ineffective, we would probably decrease her medication slowly. We would also inquire about symptoms of depression that might be affecting her schoolwork and causing pseudo-seizures. If the episodes continue despite counseling, we would need to observe an episode and the simultaneous electroencephalogram to see if the episode in question is accompanied by electrical discharge from the brain. Video-EEG monitoring (see Chapter 7) can, at times, be crucial in separating true seizures from pseudo-seizures. An EEG taken during a seizure will virtually always reveal an abnormality. EEG abnormalities found between episodes do not mean that the episodes in question were seizures.

It is important to remember that a child may have true seizures *and* pseudo-seizures. It is vital to know *which is which* so that medication can be adjusted to control any true seizures and psychological counseling initiated to eliminate the pseudo-seizures.

## The Physician's Evaluation

The child who *clearly has had a seizure* needs an appropriate evaluation. Tests that will help determine the cause of the seizure may be necessary (see Chapter 3). If the seizure has been provoked by an acute disturbance of the brain, such as infection or trauma, extensive evaluation may not be needed.

The child who *clearly has not had a seizure* may not need those tests.

*When the physician is uncertain, multiple tests may still be unnecessary since no test will tell you definitely if the event was a seizure or not. Careful observation, watching, and waiting—"Tincture of Time"—is often the best approach.*

- Almost 10 percent of all individuals will have a single seizure at some time in their lives.
- 50 to 75 percent of those who have one seizure will *never* have a second seizure.

For such reasons, it is not necessary for you or your physician to be overly concerned about the future just because your child has had one episode, even if that episode was a seizure.

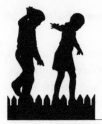

# 3. How We Evaluate and Think about a First Seizure

Since a seizure may be the sign of an acute disturbance of the nervous system, every child with a first seizure or suspected seizure should be seen immediately by a physician, who will search for a cause that may require urgent treatment.

The first thing your physician will want to know is if your child has a fever. The causes of a seizure in a child who has a fever may be quite different from the causes in a child who has none (Table 3.1).

## Febrile Seizures

❏ **The car screeches to a stop at the emergency room entrance. The mother rushes in with a small infant in her arms. "I thought my baby was dying," she sobs. "I was holding him and giving him his bottle, and all of a sudden he felt very warm to me, like he had a fever. Then his eyes rolled back in his head, he got stiff and started to jerk all over. I gave him mouth-to-mouth resuscitation, and then the jerking stopped. We just got in the car and rushed over. He's sleeping now. Is he going to be all right?"**

Most first seizures in a child less than five years of age will be what are called "febrile seizures." Seizures brought on by fever are the most common seizures of childhood and occur in 3 to 4 percent of children. Uncommon during a child's early months, they reach their peak at about eighteen months and are, in general, outgrown by the time a child is five years old. When a young child has a seizure *and* a fever, it is

**Table 3.1   Potential Causes of a First Seizure**

**With fever**
  Febrile seizure
  Meningitis (viral, bacterial)
  Encephalitis (viral)

**Without fever**
  Chemical imbalance (dehydration, excess fluids, calcium, magnesium)
  Trauma
  Tumor
  Vascular malformation, stroke

*Note:* More than 50% of first seizures in children are of unknown cause. Also, causes vary with the child's age.

urgent that he be seen by his physician to be certain that this seizure is not due to *meningitis,* an infection in or around the brain caused by bacteria or by viruses, or encephalitis, an inflammation within the brain itself that is usually the consequence of a virus. Bacterial meningitis in the past was a killer of young children, but now, with modern antibiotics *and* with early diagnosis, most children with meningitis can recover without disability. Most viral infections of the brain are mild and do not need to be treated; for the few severe viral encephalitic infections, treatments are being developed.

When your child is seen by your physician, the doctor will, of course, want to take a careful history and perform a careful physical and neurologic examination. The physician will look for the cause of the fever in the ears, throat, perhaps the urine, and he may want to check the blood count. He will consider meningitis and, depending on the child's age and how sick he looks, may consider a lumbar puncture (spinal tap) to check for infection in the fluid around the brain and spinal cord. A spinal tap sounds frightening, but it is an easy and virtually risk-free procedure in children.

*The child who has a first seizure with a fever does not necessarily need special x-rays or brain scans.*

Fever lowers the brain's threshold for seizures and thus may provoke them. Indeed, as noted earlier, a seizure can be induced in anyone if the temperature is sufficiently high. Young children have a lower seizure threshold anyway, and thus are more susceptible to a seizure when a rapidly rising fever further lowers this already low threshold. This is the reason why such seizures tend to occur in young children. The threshold gradually increases over the first years of life as the brain becomes more mature, which is why these infants and young children outgrow the tendency to febrile seizures as they grow older. Febrile seizures are very uncommon after age five or six.

Susceptibility to febrile seizures appears to have a genetic base. Such seizures tend to occur in certain families.

These three factors—the lower threshold of the infant (ages three months to two or three years), the height and rapidity of rise of the fever, and the genetic threshold—all three in combination may lower the seizure threshold sufficiently to cause a seizure. A higher fever or more rapid rise in fever in an infant without a family history of seizures may be enough to trigger a seizure; a lower fever in an infant with such a family history may be enough. In an older child, whose threshold is higher, a high fever may be sufficient with a family history of febrile or afebrile (nonfebrile) seizures, but insufficient to trigger a seizure without a family history of seizures.

The first seizure with fever can be terrifying to a parent. Occasionally the seizure may be mild and brief (no more than slight slumping and loss of consciousness, or a rolling of the eyes back in the head), but often there is stiffening, a jerking, and loss of consciousness. Nine out of ten febrile seizures last only a few minutes, usually fewer than ten, but even they seem to last a lifetime to parents who have never seen a seizure before and who believe that their child is choking, or swallowing his tongue, or even dying.

### What Should You Do during a Seizure?

A child who is having a seizure should be placed on her side and protected from sharp objects. Tight clothing should be loosened.

- Do not try to put anything in your child's mouth—she will not swallow her tongue.
- Do not restrain your child's movements.

Most of these seizures will stop on their own in a few minutes. If one seizure lasts more than ten to fifteen minutes, or if the seizure is repeated two or more times, call an ambulance or take your child to the emergency room yourself or to your doctor's office. If the child is still having a seizure, the physician will want to give medication to be sure that the seizure stops promptly.

The child does not *necessarily* have to stay in a hospital, just because she has a fever and has had a seizure. The decision about hospitalization is a judgment to be left to you and your physician.

Most children with febrile seizures will recover from the seizure very quickly (within an hour) and can usually return home. Children with meningitis or encephalitis may have a varying course—from a mild illness to one that is severe or even fatal—and probably will need to stay in the hospital for a period of time.

## After the Seizure Is Over

If the seizure has stopped, the physician will want to find the cause of the fever and hence of the seizure. Because it is the physician's first responsibility to assure that the fever and seizure are not caused by meningitis, he will have examined the child. If the child is more than two to three years of age, clinical examination can determine this. If the child is under one year of age or if there is any question about meningitis, a spinal tap should be performed to rule out the presence of this infection.

Your doctor will probably recommend other tests to search for the source of the fever that triggered the seizure. In the young child with a first seizure with a fever, tests for other causes of the seizure are rarely helpful, however. If the child has recovered from the seizure and is running around the doctor's office, as is true after most febrile seizures, further testing with scans and EEGs is rarely helpful. The physician can best try to calm your own fears by giving you information about seizures of this kind.

## Questions You Will Ask

You will have many questions about febrile seizures, among them these:

### "Will he have more seizures?"

Only 25 to 30 percent of children who have had one febrile seizure will ever have another. If the first febrile seizure occurs in the first year of life, *and* if there is a family history of febrile seizures or epilepsy, *and* if the child's seizure has been long or complicated, then that child may have a high chance (>80%) of having another febrile seizure. If the child has none of these risk factors, the chances of recurrence may be as low as one in ten.

However, a child who has a second seizure has about four chances in ten of having a third, and after a third, also four in ten chances of having a fourth. But only nine in a hundred children with febrile seizures do have three or more.

### *"What will happen if he does have another?"*

Nothing is likely to happen to your child as a result of the febrile seizure.

- There is *no* evidence that recurrent febrile seizures damage the brain.
- Children who have febrile seizures *do not* develop mental retardation as a consequence of the seizures.
- These children do not develop cerebral palsy as a result of these seizures.
- There is *no* evidence that these children have an increased chance of learning disabilities.

Children who have one, two, or even three or more febrile seizures grow up just like children who have never had such seizures. Virtually the *only* consequence of a febrile seizure is an increased chance of having another febrile seizure.

### *"What about a seizure that lasts more than twenty minutes? Will it recur?"*

Only one in ten febrile seizures lasts more than twenty minutes, and most of those prolonged seizures are the initial seizure only. A child who has had a prolonged first febrile seizure is no more likely to have a prolonged second seizure than if the first seizure were short.

### *"Can't these seizures be prevented?"*

Certain medications can markedly decrease the chance of another febrile seizure, but there are risks as well as benefits. You will have to weigh the risks of the medicine and the benefits of avoiding another febrile seizure against the risks of having another seizure.

Phenobarbital is the most effective medication for preventing recurrence of febrile seizures, although ineffective when the child already has the fever. If it is given on a daily basis in sufficient quantities, there will be a marked decrease in the chance of another seizure. The amount of phenobarbital in the blood should be checked periodically to be sure that there is enough.

### *"What about side effects of medication?"*

Phenobarbital produces side effects, however, especially in infants and young children. Many children (20–40 percent) who take phenobarbital will become hyperactive, or will develop behavior problems or disturbances of sleep. For more than half, the side effects are sufficiently severe so that the phenobarbital has to be discontinued. Even more important, there is also evidence that phenobarbital may decrease intelligence and affect learning.

Unfortunately, there is no current treatment without risks of side effects. Medications such as phenytoin (Dilantin) and carbamazepine (Tegretol) do not prevent febrile seizures. Sodium valproate (Depakene), when taken daily, is as effective as phenobarbital in preventing recurrences, but in this very young age group there is also a high risk (as high as one in 800) that sodium valproate may cause severe, even fatal, liver disease. As a consequence, we rarely recommend sodium valproate for the prevention of febrile seizures.

There is some evidence that diazepam (Valium), given by mouth or rectally when the child has a fever, decreases the chances of another febrile seizure. This may be useful if a child lives at a great distance from medical care or if there is concern about a prolonged febrile seizure. However, given intermittently like this, diazepam may cause sleepiness and irritability.

Since there is increasing information that the chances of recurrence of seizures are low, and the consequences of recurrence few, there is increasing consensus among physicians to avoid recommending any continuous medication. We only consider continuous medication in the very rare instance of a child who has many seizures with fever.

### *"What is the chance of my child's developing epilepsy?"*

Some people now consider any recurrent seizures, even two or more febrile seizures, to be epilepsy. However, most people think of epilepsy as recurrent seizures that are not provoked by fever. Febrile seizures do not cause epilepsy. The chance of epilepsy developing is slightly higher in a child who has had a febrile seizure than in one who has not, but not much greater (see Table 3.2).

Of children who have had a febrile seizure, more than ninety-eight out of 100 will never have epilepsy.

**Table 3.2    Risks Associated with Febrile Seizures**

| Type of risk | % Risk |
| --- | --- |
| Risk of: | |
| Mental retardation | No greater than |
| Cerebral palsy | in children without |
| Learning problems | febrile seizures |
| Death | |
| Risk of another febrile seizure | |
| After 1 seizure | 30–40 |
| After 2 seizures | 40.0 |
| After 3 seizures | 40.0 |
| Risk of epilepsy | |
| If there were no febrile seizures | 0.5 |
| If there was 1 febrile seizure | 2.0 |
| Risk of epilepsy after 1 febrile seizure | |
| 0 risk factors | 0.1 |
| 1 risk factor | 2.5 |
| 3 risk factors | 5–10.0 |

*Note:* Risk Factors: Seizures prolonged >15 minutes, one-sided, or 2 or more seizures during the same day; parent or brother or sister with epilepsy; neurologic disorder or developmental delay.

The "risk factors" for later epilepsy developing in a child who has had a single febrile seizure are:

• If the first febrile seizure is prolonged (more than fifteen minutes), if the seizure was one-sided or focal, or if there were two or more seizures during that initial episode;
• If there is a family history of epilepsy;
• If the child has a neurologic disorder, such as cerebral palsy, or if his development had been delayed before the seizure.

A child who has a febrile seizure but none of these risk factors has approximately one chance in 100 of later epilepsy. A child with one factor has a 2.5 percent chance, and a child with two or more risk factors has a 5 to 10 percent chance of epilepsy.

Thus, in the worst situation, a child who has all three risk factors would have only one chance in ten of epilepsy.

*"Isn't there anything that can be done to reduce even these small risks?"*

There is no evidence that the risks of epilepsy increase, even if your child has more febrile seizures. There is also no evidence that placing your child on medication after a febrile seizure will reduce the risks of later epilepsy.

## Evaluation of the Child with a First Seizure without Fever

Now, let's talk about the evaluation of a child who has had a first seizure *without fever*.

If your child clearly has had a seizure, your first question, and indeed that of your physician, is "Why? What caused it?" While laboratory tests neither prove nor disprove that your child has had a seizure, they can, at times, be very helpful in searching for a cause and in predicting the likelihood of further seizures.

Since a seizure is the result of a disturbance of normal brain function and since there can be many different types of disturbances, there are many different causes of seizures.

One type of disturbance is acute, usually only temporary, and while capable of causing a single seizure (a single provoked seizure), rarely causes recurrent seizures. Since some of these—causes such as infection or trauma—could require urgent treatment, your physician will concentrate on them at the time of your child's first seizure.

*Most first seizures without fever are of unknown cause.*

While not knowing a cause for the seizure is frustrating, the diagnosis of an *idiopathic* seizure (a seizure of unknown cause) is the best possible diagnosis for your child. A diagnosis of idiopathic seizure is an occasion for considerable optimism. It means that your doctor hasn't found a serious cause. More than half of first seizures are idiopathic. Idiopathic seizures are likely to be completely controlled with medication and are likely to be outgrown. If there is a single such seizure, your child does not have epilepsy.

Evaluation of a child who has no fever depends on many factors: the age of the child, the type of seizure, how soon after the seizure the child is seen, and whether the child has returned to normal. The frequency of various causes of seizures changes with the age of the patient (see Fig. 3.1). After taking a careful history, the physician will look for general physical abnormalities. Abnormalities of the heart's rhythm or rate may lead to a lack of oxygen to the brain, other heart disease to strokes

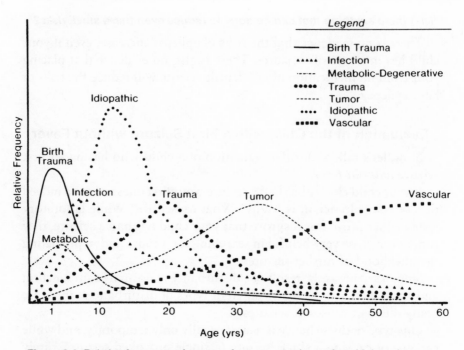

**Figure 3.1.** Relative frequency of causes of new onset seizures from birth to sixty years.

and seizures. Lung problems can cause brain infection. High blood pressure can cause seizures, as can acute or chronic kidney disease. Some birthmarks provide evidence of problems in the brain that may cause seizures, so your physician will look carefully at your child's skin. Brain tumors and cancer are rare causes of seizures in children. Your doctor will also want to concentrate on the child's neurologic function and on your child's development to detect any *new* neurologic abnormality that might suggest a stroke, infection, or tumor requiring treatment; to verify that there is *no* abnormality; or to document old neurologic abnormalities for comparison with future examinations.

A careful neurologic exam does not necessarily require a neurologist. If your physician is concerned about some of the findings or discovers suspicious abnormalities, he may want to refer you to a specialist, a child neurologist.

"You mean that's all there is? You tell us our son has had a seizure and you're only going to talk to us and examine Peter. Aren't you going to do any tests?" you ask. The physician's appropriate response to that question is, "There is no laboratory test for a seizure. The diagnosis of a seizure depends on your description of what happened."

Some tests can be of help in looking for a cause of the seizure. Certain tests help the physician rule out other peculiar episodes that simulate seizures. He may want to do an electrocardiogram if he is concerned about abnormalities of heart rate or rhythm. He may order blood tests if he suspects anemia, diabetes, or other chemical problems. But the diagnosis of a seizure itself can only be made by direct observation of the spell by a physician or by his careful interpretation of the observations of others.

The most common tests performed when a child has had a seizure are an EEG and a CT or MRI scan. Some people think that a brain wave test, an electroencephalogram (EEG), will diagnose epilepsy. But an EEG does not diagnose a seizure unless a seizure occurs *during* the EEG. The EEG may, however, be very helpful in suggesting the appropriate treatment of children with seizures. A CT scan or MRI may, in the proper circumstances, be useful in searching for the cause of the seizure, but a brain scan does not diagnose epilepsy itself. Nor does it rule it out. Although they may be useful in determining the cause of a seizure, both EEGs and scans can be normal in the child who has had a seizure and either or both may be abnormal in an otherwise normal child who has not and never will have a seizure. A detailed discussion of these tests is in Chapter 7.

Just as after a first febrile seizure, after a first afebrile seizure you will have many questions: "Will it recur?" "Can it be prevented?" "What are the risks of prevention?" The remainder of the book will address these questions for you.

Your first questions may be, "Will he have more seizures?" "Can't they be prevented?" Yes, there is some risk of another seizure occurring. There are medications that may prevent further seizures, but they entail risks. Therefore, let's begin by discussing risks and benefits.

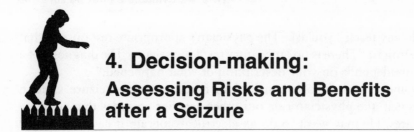

# 4. Decision-making:
## Assessing Risks and Benefits after a Seizure

**"When are you going to start Frank on medication? What are its side effects?"**

**"Now that Sarah has had a seizure, how long before I can allow her to ride her bike again?"**

**"Billy was going to go on a trip out west this summer. Should I put down the deposit? Will he be able to go?"**

Life is full of risks and benefits. We take risks for ourselves and for our children every day. Although no one would ever do it, the safest place to raise a child is in a padded cell. In that cell the child cannot be injured when he falls down, tumbles from a tree, or crosses in front of a car. Your child will be safe! But you will be sorry. Clearly, a child raised without risk would be a very abnormal child. Living, therefore, is best seen as a series of assessments of the relative importance of risks and benefits. Making decisions about which risks (costs) to take for which benefits is what we all do subconsciously all the time.

Risk-benefit analysis involves weighing the good against the bad. On the good side of the scale, we calculate the chance of a benefit and worth of the benefit. A small chance of winning a large amount of money in the lottery may be "worth it" and outweigh the risk involved in losing a small amount of money. Worth has different meanings in different situations and to different people. Achieving "worth" or "winning" always involves some risks and consequences that must be weighed against the potential benefits.

Medicine is a series of risk-benefit analyses. In the past, physicians tended to do all of the analysis for you and recommended what you should do—whether your child should take medication and what medications he should take. This is much easier for the parent, and perhaps for the doctor as well since it doesn't involve as much time and discussion. With the advent of a more medically sophisticated public, however, the patient and the family are, and should be, more closely involved in the decision-making process. The physician will still weigh the risks and the benefits and make recommendations on the basis of his assessment, but you as parent should weigh them as well. The risks of what he recommends are *your* risks (or your child's), not his, and the benefits that accrue, accrue to *you or your child*. You may evaluate the worth of the benefits or the consequences of the risks differently from your physician.

Some decisions in medicine are clear and easy, others are more difficult. If your physician thinks your child has appendicitis, not operating could lead to a ruptured appendix and infection resulting in, at least, a severe illness and, at worst, death. The risks of operating are small with modern anesthesia, but there is a small risk of death and of infection with any operation. Comparing the risks of surgery with those of not operating, virtually anyone would recommend surgery. But suppose the signs of appendicitis are not clear and there is only some tenderness in her abdomen. Your doctor might postpone surgery because the risks of an operation might be greater than the risks of waiting. As the child is observed, the time may come when the risks of waiting outweigh the risks and consequences of surgery.

As we talk about the risks and benefits of the decisions you will now have to make about your child and her seizure management, keep in mind that:

• There will be risks and benefits to each decision you make *or don't make;*
• These risks and benefits will vary greatly in their consequences and in the magnitude of the consequence, both good and bad;
• The risks and benefits are *yours and your child's,* not your physician's;
• Frequently there are no "correct" or "incorrect" decisions, as

far as we can see. Different people will come to different decisions. However, there are always consequences to whatever decision is made or not made and they must be assessed in advance as far as is possible.

No one can accurately predict the future. Consequences are not always foreseeable. Therefore, you and your physician must always make the best decision possible without feeling guilty if things don't work out the way you planned.

## Whether or Not to Use Medicine

The first decision you face may be whether to treat your child after a first seizure.

At one time, physicians believed that a single seizure was the first sign of epilepsy, and that a person who had one seizure would inevitably have more. Therefore, after the first seizure they prescribed medication to prevent the recurrence that was "bound" to occur. Today, we, like many other physicians, do not believe this.

We have learned that after a single seizure of unknown cause the chance of recurrence may range from 10 to 50 percent, depending on a number of factors. Children with a first seizure and a normal EEG appear to have a low risk of recurrence. Children with an abnormal EEG may have a much higher risk of recurrence.

### "Should my child begin taking daily medication after her first seizure?"

What are the chances of another seizure recurring in your child? If her chances of having another seizure were 10 to 15 percent, would you consider this a high chance or a low one? The consequences of a second seizure will depend on the child's age and the type of seizure. The consequences of a seizure could be great for older adolescents or adults if, for example, they are driving a car. The consequences of prohibiting driving are great for this age group. The younger child faces no such consequences. The consequences of everyday activities, therefore, vary with age. The toddler is unlikely to be climbing a tree, while the older child may be climbing when a seizure occurs. Risks and consequences vary dramatically with age, with activities, and also personality, as well as many other factors. Since the consequences will happen to you and your child, you (and sometimes your child) will have to be the one to evaluate their significance.

Medication is usually started to decrease the chance of another seizure. But does medication do this? It is widely believed that medication is effective in preventing seizures, and indeed, it is clearly effective in people who have frequent seizures. It is not as clear that it prevents a second seizure in a child who has had only one. A number of studies suggest that the risk of a second seizure is just as great for the child who is placed on medication as for the child who is not. Therefore, whether medication is effective in this situation remains a matter of debate.

You might want to try medicine anyway *if* it involved no risks or negative consequences.

Unfortunately, however, there *are* both risks and consequences. The cost of medication can be significant for some families. Every medication has side effects (risks and consequences). The "cost" in terms of side effects can be substantial. You have to evaluate the costs and benefits for your child.

*"I don't even know the names of the medicines! How do you expect me to know and evaluate the risks of their side effects?"*

*Ask your doctor about the medicines.* We will discuss the various medications and their side effects in detail later. But here is one example of decision-making with one medication commonly used in children, phenobarbital. Phenobarbital is a very safe anticonvulsant, but a frequent and often ignored side effect in children is a negative effect on learning or on behavior. Of young children who take this medicine, 20 to 40 percent will become hyperactive, or incur personality or sleep problems. When carefully evaluated, there may also be some subtle effects on the child's intelligence and ability to learn.

To decide whether or not to start phenobarbital, it would be useful to list the pros and cons of the decision. Such a list might look something like this:

*If you start your child on medication there is:*

- a 30 percent chance of the child's having another seizure;
- a 10 percent chance of a rash developing that will require discontinuing medication and a small chance of a severe allergic reaction;
- a 20 to 40 percent chance of hyperactivity or behavior problems developing from the medication;
- an unknown chance of learning problems developing.

*If you decide not to start your child on medication there is:*

• a 30 percent chance of having another seizure;
• a 0 percent chance of a rash or a severe allergic reaction developing;
• a 0 percent chance of hyperactivity or behavioral and learning problems developing.

*Thus, after a single seizure, it does not appear that medication substantially reduces the chance of another seizure and, indeed, phenobarbital, for one, like other anticonvulsant medications, produces its own risks. Are there benefits associated with starting phenobarbital that outweigh the risks?*

There are no clear benefits to the child; one benefit may be your sense of confidence that he will not now have another seizure. The use of medication after a first seizure is not necessarily responsible for your child not having another seizure since seven out of ten children who have had only one seizure will never have another one *whether or not* they are treated. The use of medication in children who have repeated seizures (epilepsy) can, however, have very different and clear benefits.

Each anticonvulsant medication has its own risks and side effects. Some risks are greater than those of phenobarbital in certain children, some are less. Whenever a new medication is considered, one must weigh the risks and benefits of that particular medication.

We, at Johns Hopkins, usually do not recommend starting a child on medication after the first seizure. Other physicians may and do come to different conclusions. Parents may weigh the risks and benefits in different fashions. Every child's situation is unique. Therefore, there is no *single* "correct" answer to the question, "Should we start a child on medication after his first seizure?"

We have discussed the considerations regarding treatment of the child after a first "big" seizure. "Smaller" staring seizures are rarely recognized after only one spell has occurred, and, therefore, they are usually treated when recognized.

## Decisions about Everyday Life

We have discussed the advantages and disadvantages of raising your child in a padded cell. Once you allow your child out you will have to assess the risks and benefits of most of his daily activities. For example:

### *"Can my child still ride his bike?"*

To help you assess the answer, we would have to ask, "How old is the child?" "How frequently does he have seizures?" "Does he have a warning of the seizure?" "How reliably would he respond to that warning?" "How much does he ride his bike?" "How important is bike riding to him?"

You would have to assess how great are the chances of his being injured on the bike. There are substantial risks to any child of being injured while bike riding. Are they much greater now? Thinking carefully about your answers to these questions will enable you to be protective, but not overprotective. Perhaps you can be appropriately protective by insisting that he wear his helmet that has been sitting in the closet.

### *"Can my child swim?"*

We were recently asked to comment about a lawsuit against a physician who had not prohibited his patient with epilepsy from swimming. The child had drowned, as do a number of children who swim. It was not clear that this child had had a seizure at that time. Thinking about whether your child should be allowed to swim involves asking many of the same questions we asked about bike riding. "How old is the child?" "How frequently does he have seizures?" "How important is swimming?" "How well will he be supervised?" Every child who swims should be supervised. The child whose seizures are not frequent should clearly be well supervised. But, if well-supervised, should he be prohibited from swimming? These individualized decisions will be dependent upon your analysis of the risks and benefits.

Similar questions can be asked about allowing your child to go out and play, stay at another child's house, climb a tree, go on trips or go to camp, and drive a car.

We permit normal children to take risks. We do not want to shelter a child who has seizures from *all* risks. Taking risks is part of the growing process. We want simply to shelter that child from the *increased risk* associated with a seizure recurrence. But this sheltering must be accomplished at an acceptable cost.

# 5. What to Do If Your Child Has a Second Big Seizure

**"He almost died!" "He stopped breathing and turned blue." "He swallowed his tongue!" "I almost had a heart attack, I was so upset." "I just screamed!" "I called the ambulance, but it took them forever to get here." "I didn't know what to do!"**

Remember, more than two-thirds of children (and adults) who have one big seizure *never* have another one. If your child does have another what you should do is to stay calm!

**"Easy for you to say," you reply. "You've seen a lot of these things. I thought my child was going to die. How can I do nothing? He's my child!"**

Certainly, staying calm is the most difficult thing to do. It is easy for the physician or the nurse to recommend, but it's not easy to do, not even for doctors and nurses. Perhaps the most frightening thing about a big seizure is that there is little the observer or parent can do—or should do (see Table 5.1).

The stiffness at the start of a "big" tonic-clonic seizure is called the tonic phase (see page 64). This is when all of the body's muscles are contracting together. The child arches his back, and since the muscles of the chest are contracted as well, the child is essentially holding his breath. He does turn somewhat blue. In a sense, he *has* stopped breathing. But this phase *will* end! The child will not die; his heart has not stopped; you do *not* need to do CPR. The body has a protective

**Table 5.1  What to Do for a Person during a Major Seizure**

STAY CALM

**During the seizure:**
  • Do not put anything in the mouth
  • Do not restrain your child
  • Do not call an ambulance (unless the seizure continues for more than 10
      minutes)
  • Do try to lay him on his side
  • Do put something soft (coat, pillow) under his head
  • Do loosen tight clothing around his neck
  • Do remove sharp objects—chair, table, etc.—from the immediate area

**After the seizure:**
  • Do stay with him until he is awake and alert
  • Do be comforting and reassuring
  • Do allow him to go back to his activities if he's all right

mechanism built in to prevent damage. If the oxygen gets low enough, the body will usually stop the seizure long before the decreased oxygen can permanently damage brain cells.

*There is nothing you can do during this tonic phase to get rid of the stiffness or to make your child breathe.* Mouth-to-mouth resuscitation will not work since the patient's chest will not expand.

## What Should You Do?

  • *You should* turn the child on his side so that the secretions in the mouth, the saliva, can run out rather than running back into the windpipe;
  • *You should* loosen clothing around the neck so that it does not further impair the child's breathing;
  • *You should* clear things from around him, so that when the clonic, jerking phase of the seizure starts, the child does not bang himself against a chair leg or sharp edges of a table.
  • *You should,* if possible, put a soft object, such as a pillow or a shirt, under his head so that his head does not bang against the floor.

This tonic phase seems to last a long time, but in reality it rarely lasts more than thirty seconds to a minute or so.

The next phase of a big seizure is the clonic phase in which the muscles jerk rhythmically. This is the violent phase of a seizure. There is *nothing* you can or should do during this phase, either. Restraining the child does not help, because the jerks continue anyway. Unless the patient is jerking against some sort of hard object, he will not hurt himself. *You can* gently support the child on the floor, but you cannot stop the jerking. The jerking is not hurting the child; he will not remember it. But it is very frustrating for the observer, particularly a parent, to stand by and just watch.

The jerking (clonic) phase of the seizure usually will last up to several minutes. In an unusual seizure, the clonic phase may last five or (rarely) ten minutes—what seems a lifetime.

## When Should You Call for Help or an Ambulance?

ONLY IF THIS CLONIC PHASE LASTS TEN OR FIFTEEN MINUTES (some say more than five minutes by the clock) IS IT ADVISABLE TO CALL AN AMBULANCE. Virtually *all* seizures will have ceased before this time, well before the ambulance arrives. The jerking stops by gradually slowing down. Eventually the child relaxes. He often lets out a deep breath and then goes into a very deep sleep. The seizure is over. The brain is "resting." At that point, there is nothing the ambulance crew, physicians, or the emergency room can or needs to do.

Only if the seizure lasts ten to fifteen minutes is it reasonable to call an ambulance. Why call then? Because *if* the clonic seizure *is* still continuing when the ambulance finally arrives, *then* the ambulance personnel should take the child to the emergency room. It takes a few minutes to get the child on the stretcher and five to ten minutes to transport him to the emergency room. *If the child is still having a clonic seizure when he reaches the hospital, then the emergency room staff may want to give an injection to stop the seizure.* Approximately thirty minutes or more will have elapsed from the start of the seizure. That is the time when medical intervention to stop the seizure is desirable.

The timing discussed above assumes that you live in an urban setting, near an ambulance and a hospital. If you live in a more rural or inaccessible setting, it is desirable to reach a physician's office in about that same time.

A generalized tonic-clonic seizure lasting more than thirty minutes is defined as status epilepticus and will be discussed at greater length (Chapter 10). Such a seizure, lasting more than thirty minutes, *begins* to cause changes in the brain that look as if they *might* cause permanent brain damage should the seizure and these changes continue. More recent information suggests that even prolonged seizures rarely damage the brain. Rather, these studies show, it is the *cause* of the seizure—the meningitis, low blood sugar level, head trauma—which is the real cause of the permanent damage, not the seizure itself. However, we still recommend that a child with a long seizure be taken to a hospital emergency room to make sure that the seizure stops in a reasonable period of time.

As noted, as the seizure stops the child usually lets out a deep sigh and goes into a deep sleep, the post-ictal period. It is as if the brain is resting from its overexertion. The length of this post-ictal sleep will vary, depending on the duration of the seizure. It may last anywhere from ten to fifteen minutes up to an hour or two. After a short period of time, the child can be aroused but often is confused and prefers to go back to sleep. There is no reason not to let him sleep. This sleep is a healthy recovery phase.

On rare occasions, the patient may have a second seizure while still in this sleepy, post-ictal state. Serial seizures (one after the other without the patient waking up in between) is also termed status epilepticus. When this pattern occurs, the patient should also be taken to the emergency room so that these serial seizures can be stopped. They indicate that the brain is very irritable and may require medication to decrease this irritability.

**"Is there anything else I could do during the seizure? Shouldn't I put something in my child's mouth to keep him from biting his tongue?"**

The answer is, "No, you should not." Unfortunately, in many generalized seizures, the patient may bite his tongue. But putting something in the mouth is difficult. Prying the mouth open to put in a spoon or a stick is more likely to break a tooth. If, by chance, someone does have his mouth open early in the seizure, you could put a handkerchief or a shirt sleeve or something soft between the teeth to prevent biting of the tongue. Unfortunately, most people clench their teeth at the start of the seizure. *Never put your finger in the person's mouth because it can be badly bitten.*

**"What about mouth-to-mouth resuscitation. Will this help?"**

*No!* The patient will breathe on his or her own. Plus, during the seizure, your mouth-to-mouth resuscitation cannot get air into the lungs.

It is hard to watch somebody have a seizure and frustrating not to be able to intervene, to stop this terrible thing, not to be able to help. But the best thing you can do is to remain calm. By staying calm, others around you are more likely to remain calm, and when your child wakes up, often confused, he will be surrounded by a less hysterical, more supportive environment.

*"What about the child who doesn't have tonic-clonic seizures, but has seizures where he wanders around confused, picking at things, and could injure himself? What should I do during one of those?"*

During this type of seizure, what is called a "complex partial seizure," the patient *is* confused and not really aware of what he is doing or of his environment. He is likely to misunderstand and misinterpret things during this foggy state. If the child is wandering around, try and be protective. You shouldn't try to restrain him. The myths about people being aggressive during these seizures come from the child's misunderstanding and misinterpretation of what is happening and what is being done to him. If people try to restrain the child who is in this confused state, he may misunderstand the motivation and fight back. Rather, you should be protective, reassuring, and try to direct him away from dangerous objects or from hurting himself. This is perhaps all you can do. Confused ictal and post-ictal states may last several minutes; occasionally the post-ictal confusion lasts five to ten or even fifteen minutes. Again, only if this state lasts for a long period of time, more than fifteen minutes, is it necessary to bring the child to the emergency room or a physician's office, where, if it continues, the physician might want to use an injection to stop the spell.

In conclusion, what should you do? *In most cases, don't call the ambulance.* It's not needed and won't be of any help. And yet when a child, even one who has had previous seizures, has a seizure in school, the ambulance often is called. Discourage this. It is not only expensive but usually useless. Educating the teachers, school nurses, camp directors, and others who might come in contact with your child that the seizure will be over shortly and that your child will be all right is perhaps the best thing you can do both for yourself and for your child. It is as effective and far cheaper than calling the ambulance.

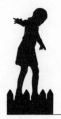

# 6. The Kinds of Seizure and Where They Arise in the Brain

Since episodic electrical events can occur in different areas of the brain, the types of seizures that they produce will differ depending on what area is affected.

## The Many Types of Seizure

❑ You heard a loud noise and ran to Johnny's room. Your son was stiff, his back was arched, he didn't seem to be breathing and he was turning blue. Then he started shaking violently, and he was foaming at the mouth. Your first thought was that he was about to die!

❑ Mary was sitting with you at the dinner table when suddenly she stopped eating and stared into space. You called her, but she didn't respond, and you had to call her several times. "Why does she daydream so often?" you wondered.

❑ William comes running to you with a frightened look on his face. He is pale and then has a glassy look to his eyes. You call him, but he doesn't respond. You notice that he is smacking his lips and fumbling with his clothes. Then as you hold him, he stiffens and begins to shake violently.

❑ Trina began to have jerking at the corner of her mouth. "It's just a habit," your doctor said, but it's gotten worse. Now the jerking is there all the time and sometimes it spreads to involve the whole side of her face.

All of these are seizures, and yet each differs. Each may require a different evaluation by your physician. Each may require different medication. Each may have a different outcome. The type of seizure depends largely on where in the brain it starts and on the direction and speed of the spread of the electrical activity.

Seizures are divided into two major groups, "partial seizures" and "generalized seizures." "Partial seizures" (simple or complex), those that begin focally—that is, in one place—are also called "focal" or "local" seizures. It is important to identify partial seizures because, since they begin focally, there may well be a specific problem in that area of the brain, one that may need special attention. The physician looks for a scar, a tangle of blood vessels, or a tumor as the cause of such seizures. If focal seizures cannot be controlled with medication, then surgery can be considered. "Generalized seizures," on the other hand, seem to start all over the brain at once. We are unable to detect either by clinical signs or symptoms, and sometimes not even from the EEG, where this widespread electrical activity begins.

Partial seizures have implications different from generalized seizures. Since they start in one particular area of the brain, they may require special evaluation; they may also require the use of particular medications or other therapy. To help the physician determine the proper course, it is important, as noted earlier, for you to focus carefully on the very onset of the seizure and its progression so you may be able to describe it precisely to him.

When seizures start focally in a particular area of the brain, and when they spread slowly enough, in seconds or minutes as in William's seizure, so that their onset is experienced and witnessed or remembered, this onset is the "aura" or warning, the warning that bigger things are coming.

How do focal seizures spread to become generalized? Why don't all focal seizures spread? What contains a focal seizure? If we knew the answers to these questions, we would understand far more about epilepsy and be better able to prevent or limit seizures than we are. But we have few answers at the present time. Generalized seizures that appear to start in all parts of the brain simultaneously have no identifiable focal onset. We do not understand their anatomy. It does not make sense for the whole brain spontaneously and suddenly to experience a disruption. Nevertheless, in generalized seizures this is what appears to occur, causing disruptions like staring, stiffening, or shaking.

## Special Terms Used to Describe the Phases of a Seizure

Physicians commonly use certain special terms to describe parts of a seizure, terms referred to briefly early in this book: "aura," "ictus," and "post-ictal."

*Aura.* An "aura" is simply the start of a partial seizure. The frightened feeling or look William experienced is called an aura if it precedes a bigger seizure. If the feeling is all that William experiences, he is said to "have had an aura—a simple partial seizure." This may be the warning of an even more widespread seizure to come. If the seizure spreads within the temporal lobe and affects consciousness, then it becomes a complex partial seizure. If it spreads throughout the brain resulting in stiffening and generalized shaking, it becomes a generalized seizure. But with each seizure, the onset, which may be an abnormal smell, taste, abdominal sensation, or emotion (its focal beginning), is still called the aura.

*Ictus.* "Ictus" is the Latin word for "stroke" or "attack." Physicians sometimes use the word to mean a seizure. Thus, a simple partial seizure involving the hand, or a complex partial seizure, even a generalized seizure with loss of consciousness and jerking, could each be termed an ictus.

*Post-ictal.* "Post-ictal" means after the attack or seizure. After a person has had a seizure involving motor activity of her arm, the arm may be weak or even paralyzed for minutes or hours. This is termed a "post-ictal" paralysis, also called Todd's paralysis, after the physician who identified it. After a generalized tonic-clonic seizure, the person may go to sleep for a period. This is called the post-ictal state. After a partial complex seizure, the person may have post-ictal confusion. Each of these conditions occurs *after* the seizure is over.

Just as overexcitement and rapid synchronous firing of the neurons characterize the active phase of the seizure, so in the post-ictal phase the predominant activity of the brain is inhibitory. Neurons are less likely to fire. This effect has helped to quiet the excitability of the cortex and stop the seizure. However, because inhibition also prevents the cells from resuming their normal activity, the person is sleepy or confused or may experience a temporary paralysis.

When observers say, "This person's seizure lasted an hour," what they really mean is that the individual had a generalized tonic-clonic seizure, which may have lasted only five minutes, but that the person then slept (was in a post-ictal state) for an hour. The difference between the two is important, because there is *no* danger from the post-ictal state. That quiescent state is simply the time necessary for the brain to recover and return to its normal functioning; whereas, if the seizure (jerking) had lasted for the entire hour, that would have been considered a medical emergency.

## How Are Seizures Classified?

### The Old System: "Grand Mal" and "Petit Mal" Seizures

At one time, seizures were classified into two types: big and small—in French, *grand* and *petit*. Since seizures were bad—*mal* in French—they were classified as "grand mal" and "petit mal," terms still, unfortunately, used by many patients and by many physicians—unfortunately because they are imprecise. Many types of seizures are "big and bad," causing a patient to fall to the ground and shake. Johnny's seizure and William's seizure caused each child respectively to fall down and shake, and thus, in the old days, both would have been called grand mal seizures. We know they are different because William's seizure had a partial, or focal, beginning.

The term "grand mal" (big and bad) means different things to different people. Some people consider a seizure "big" that another, with worse seizures, might consider "small." If one person has a spell in which he just stops and stares, as Mary did, while another, like William, has a spell in which he stares, smacks his lips, and is confused, and a third, such as Trina, has jerking of the face—are these little spells all "petit mal"? They are different types of seizures, coming from different parts of the brain, with different implications of causation, requiring different evaluation, requiring different medications, and probably having differing outcomes. Thus, the terms grand mal and petit mal are now seldom used in classifying seizures.

### The New System: "Partial" and "Generalized" Seizures

An internationally accepted system of classification of seizures was adopted in 1981 (Table 6.1). This new classification separates seizures into "partial" ("simple" and "complex") and "generalized."

Partial seizures may or may not alter consciousness or awareness, depending on where they start and which structures of the brain they involve. Partial seizures that do *not* alter consciousness are called "sim-

**Table 6.1   Seizure Classification**

| International classification | "Old terms" |
| --- | --- |
| **Partial seizures** | Focal or local seizures |
| Simple partial seizures (consciousness not impaired) | |
| • With motor symptoms | Focal motor Jacksonian seizures |
| • With somatosensory symptoms | Focal sensory |
| • With autonomic symptoms | |
| • With psychic symptoms | |
| Complex partial seizures (consciousness impaired) | Psychomotor seizures Temporal lobe seizures |
| • Simple partial onset | |
| • With impairment of consciousness at onset | |
| Partial seizures that secondarily generalize | |
| **Generalized seizures** | |
| (Convulsive or non-convulsive) | |
| • Absence | Petit mal |
| Absence | |
| Atypical | |
| • Myoclonic | Minor motor |
| • Clonic seizures | Grand mal |
| • Tonic seizures | Grand mal |
| • Tonic-clonic seizures | Grand mal |
| • Atonic seizures | Akinetic, drop attacks Minor motor |

*Note:* Adapted from *Epilepsia* 22:493–95, 1981.

ple partial seizures", in the past called "focal motor" or "focal sensory" seizures. Partial seizures in which consciousness is altered or lost are called "complex partial seizures."

Generalized seizures affect the whole brain, not just one part, and they alter consciousness. In a generalized seizure, there is no obvious partial or focal onset or aura. When there is a focal onset, and the seizure progresses to involve the whole brain, it is termed a "partial seizure with secondary generalization."

Generalized seizures come in two sizes: large and small—convulsive and nonconvulsive. *Nonconvulsive* refers to alterations of consciousness but without jerking movements. *Convulsive* here means that there are muscle movements like jerking or stiffening.

## Generalized Seizures

### Absence Seizures

An absence seizure, formerly called *petit mal,* is a very special and uncommon type of seizure. It starts suddenly and without warning. The child assumes a glazed look and stares. She doesn't know what is happening and usually cannot recall things that occurred during the seizure. Occasionally, there is a little eye-blinking or head-bobbing. The episode usually lasts just seconds, occasionally as long as fifteen seconds, and ends just as abruptly as it started. When the seizure ends, the child is immediately alert. There is *no* confusion afterward. These seizures may occur *many* times a day and are often mistaken for daydreaming.

It is usually easy for the physician to produce an absence seizure in his office by making such a child take deep breaths. Usually fifteen to thirty deep breaths (hyperventilation) will produce a typical spell. (Don't worry, exercise, such as running, swimming, or bike riding, which may make someone "out of breath," does *not* produce one of these spells.)

A parent may only see a few seizures because the brain's activity must be interrupted for more than one second before a spell is apparent. Thus, very brief electrical events (less than one second in duration) are observable only on the EEG. But, in a sense, the child's awareness may be being interrupted frequently, and the child may miss some of what is going on around him.

Occasionally a person with these spells describes life "like a movie in which brief segments have been cut out." Teachers describe the child as daydreaming. Friends may call the child "spacey."

Atypical absence seizures are similar to absence seizures, but may have more pronounced motor symptoms, such as tonic or clonic spells, or may have automatisms as seen in complex partial seizures. The EEG does not have the classic three-per-second spike and wave pattern seen in simple absence seizures. Atypical absence seizures are more commonly seen in children with a damaged nervous system and are often associated with other types of seizures.

Absence seizures may superficially be confused with complex partial seizures because both involve staring. Since they both may require different treatments and have different outcomes, the differentiation may be important (see complex partial seizures below).

### Myoclonic Seizures

Myoclonic seizures (myo, meaning muscle—clonic, meaning jerk) are abrupt jerks of muscle groups. A hand may suddenly fling out, a shoulder may shrug, the foot may kick. Occasionally an entire body may jerk, as in a startle response. *All myoclonic jerks are not seizures.* Myoclonic jerks can come from the spinal cord, not just from the brain. They need not be abnormal. Normal individuals who are falling asleep may suddenly experience a jerk of the body and startle awake. This is a normal phenomenon called sleep myoclonus and is *not* a seizure.

Myoclonic seizures (formerly called minor motor seizures) may take many different forms. They probably arise, or at least the jerk arises, from deep structures in the brain stem that control posture and tone in the body.

An abrupt increase in tone in a muscle group will cause a sudden movement of that part of the body. An abrupt increase in tone in the flexor muscles will cause the body to bend forward at the waist, the head to drop down on the chest, the arms to bend at the elbow, or the knees to come up to the chest. Any or all of these movements may occur during a myoclonic jerk or during myoclonic seizures. If they occur when a child is standing, she may suddenly be thrown to the ground, perhaps hitting her face, breaking a tooth, or cutting her forehead. If the tone is suddenly increased in the extensor muscles, the head may be thrown back, the back may arch, the legs extend, and the arms stiffen. A child who is standing may be thrown backward to the ground.

*Myoclonic seizures are serious because they may be difficult to control and because they are often only one manifestation of a mixed seizure disorder commonly associated with mental retardation.*

Myoclonic seizures are like being jolted by an electric shock. They are single jolts. On rare occasions, infants and young children may experience a *series* of these jolts, sometimes even many series per day. Such a series of myoclonic jerks constitutes a special, serious form of epilepsy called "infantile spasms" (see page 108).

### Atonic Seizures

Atonic seizures, like myoclonic seizures, are sudden, single events. However, rather than a sudden increase in tone causing a movement of a joint or flexion or extension of the whole body, atonic seizures are a sudden *loss* of tone or posture. Arms, legs, or body muscles, instead of supporting the body by their tone, suddenly go limp. The body slumps or gives way. The arms may suddenly fall, the legs give way, or the body crumple to the ground.

Atonic seizures, like myoclonic seizures, probably originate in areas deep in the brain stem that control muscle tone. Since the areas that increase tone are close to those that decrease tone, children with seizures involving sudden changes in tone may have either myoclonic or atonic seizures and often both.

### Tonic-Clonic Seizures

Tonic-clonic seizures, formerly called grand mal seizures, are the sort most people think of when "seizure" is mentioned. The most memorable and frightening type of seizure to the observer, they are the most common seizure type in children, although not in adults, and despite common misconceptions are unlikely to result in brain damage or in death.

In a tonic-clonic seizure, the person initially stiffens and simultaneously loses consciousness (and thus is unaware of events). The stiffening is called the tonic phase and causes the individual to fall to the ground. The eyes "roll back in the head," the head goes back, the back arches, and the arms stiffen, as do the legs. This is similar to what happens during a myoclonic, extensor seizure, but this tonic phase of a tonic-clonic seizure happens more slowly. The extension is continued for what seems like an eternity but rarely lasts more than thirty seconds.

Since during this tonic (stiff) phase all the muscles are contracted, the chest muscles contract as well, and it is difficult for the person to breathe. He often turns somewhat blue about the lips and face (due as much to the face being flushed with the bluish blood of the veins as to the lack of oxygen). A child's saliva may cause a gurgling sound in his mouth or throat.

It is the blueness and gurgling sound that may cause observers to exclaim, "My God, he's swallowed his tongue!" This is a common misconception. A person can't swallow his tongue since it is attached to the back of the throat. "Quick, stick something in his mouth to keep him from biting his tongue!" someone else may advise, but this is bad advice. At the onset of the tonic phase of a seizure, the jaw becomes tightly clenched, and attempts to pry it open and put something in are likely to result in broken teeth.

After the tonic phase of a tonic-clonic seizure, rhythmic jerking begins. This is the clonic phase. The fists are tightly clenched, the arms repeatedly flex at the elbows and then briefly relax. The legs flex at the hip and knee joint in a similar fashion; the head may flex and then fall backwards. These movements are rhythmic and rapid, initially several per second, but then slowing. They are not the flailing movements or trembling often seen in imitation (pseudo) seizures. This rhythmic jerking seems to last forever, although only occasionally does it last more than a few minutes. Then the jerking becomes less severe and occurs at a slower rate, finally ceasing. The end of the jerking is usually accompanied by a deep sigh, after which normal breathing resumes.

The seizure is now over, but the child is not awake and will not yet respond. This post-seizure period is the post-ictal state when the brain can be thought of as "exhausted" from all its activity. In reality, the brain is quite active, but its major activity is to inhibit (stop) the cells from firing. This inhibition has brought the seizures under control.

The post-ictal period often lasts a few minutes, longer if the tonic-clonic period has been long. If left alone, the person may sleep but can be aroused and may feel tired and confused. Muscles may be sore, and the tongue may have been bitten. The best course of action for an observer at this time is to be supportive and reassuring. Allow the person to rest until he is alert and able to go his own way.

A seizure occasionally may be just the tonic (stiffening) phase described under tonic-clonic seizures. The tonic phase lasts for only a short while, usually less than a minute, and may be followed by a post-ictal sleep. A patient may on rare occasions experience a clonic seizure with the rhythmic movements previously described, but without the preceding tonic phase. Management during and after the clonic seizure is identical to that after a tonic-clonic seizure.

There is no important distinction among these last three types of seizures—tonic, clonic, and tonic-clonic—formerly called grand mal seizures. Their causes are variable, their outlooks are the same, and their management with medication is identical.

### Partial (Focal) Seizures and the Anatomy of the Brain

In order to understand partial or focal seizures and their many manifestations, it is necessary to understand something about the anatomy of the brain. Indeed, it was from a careful study of the events that occurred during partial or focal seizures that Dr. Hughlings Jackson, considered the father of modern understanding of epilepsy, first deduced the organization of the brain. He watched the slow spread of focal seizures (subsequently called Jacksonian seizures) from the finger to the hand to the arm and then to the face, and reasoned that these areas must be next to one another in the brain. The result was the identification of a continuity, the anatomy of the motor strip (Fig. 6.1).

These deductions subsequently have been confirmed by Dr. Wilder Penfield and Dr. Herbert Jasper, who, during operations to remove tissue responsible for focal epilepsy, stimulated areas of the brain with small amounts of electricity. Depending on which area was stimulated, a finger would move, a foot would jerk, the face and tongue would twitch, or a finger or lip would tingle. Even certain memories or visions would be recalled. Minute electrical stimulation is used even today to "map the brain" before a surgeon removes electrically-abnormal brain tissue so that tissue important to normal function can be identified and avoided during the surgery (see Chapter 13).

As the human brain has evolved, its "thinking and processing" parts have become greatly enlarged. This "thinking" part of the brain is the cortex. The cortex has four major sections called lobes, responsible for separate functions (Fig. 6.2A). The frontal lobes are responsible for personality and memory. The temporal lobes on the left side (in most people) control speech and on the right control subtle higher functions such as spatial recognition and music. The parietal lobes contain areas for making associations and interpreting sensations, such as the ability to recognize objects placed in the hand. The occipital lobes are the site of processing vision.

The *left* side of the brain controls movements of the *right* side of the body and receives sensation from the *right* side of the body. Thus, the left occipital lobe processes vision from things in your right field of

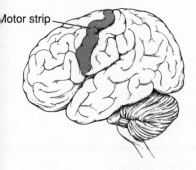

Motor strip

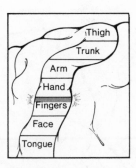

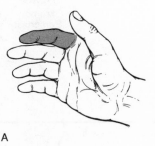

A

**Figure 6.1.** Brain, showing motor strip and progression of Jacksonian seizure. Hughlings Jackson observed the slow spread of seizures from jerking of a finger (A), to jerking of all fingers (B), to involvement of hand and wrist (C), then arm and face (D). From this spread he deduced the anatomy of the motor strip of the brain. Hence, seizures of this sort are called Jacksonian seizures.

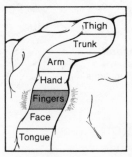

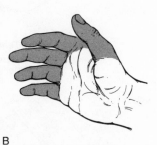

B

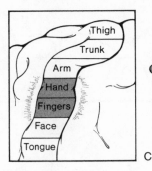

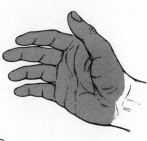

C

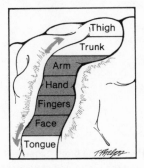

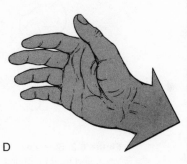

D

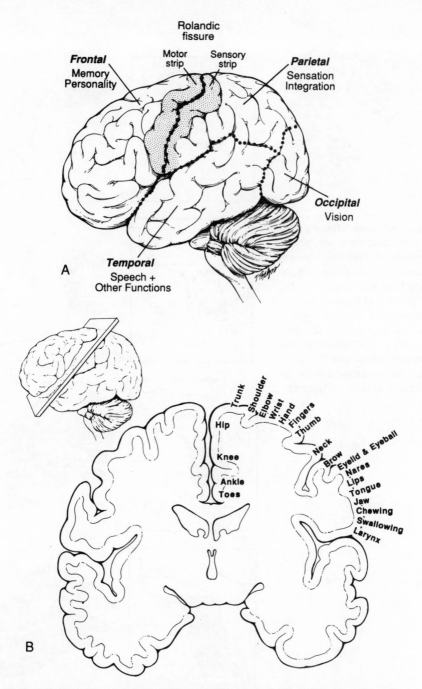

**Figure 6.2.** Side-view and slice of the brain. Side-view of a brain (A) shows the major lobes and their functions and the motor and sensory strips; a slice of the brain (B) shows location of motor and sensory functions.

**Table 6.2 Localization of Function within the Brain**

| Function | Area | Left brain | Right brain | Deficit if removed |
|---|---|---|---|---|
| Motor | Motor strip | Control of face, arm, and leg on right side of body | Control of face, arm, and leg on left side of body | Weakness (hemiparesis) of the opposite side |
| Sensory | Sensory strip | Sensation from right side of body | Sensation from left side of body | None |
| Cortical sensation | Parietal lobe | Integration of sensation from right side of body | Integration of sensation from left side of body | Inability to identify what is in hand, where hand is in space, whom hand belongs to, and so on |
| Vision | Occipital lobe | Vision to the right side of the body | Vision to the left side of the body | Lack of vision of things to one side or the other |
| Speech | Temporal lobe | Speech (on left side in 95% of right-handed people, on left side in 70% of left-handed people) | | |
| Intelligence Personality Sense of humor | Not lateralized or localized | | | |

vision, and the *right* side of the brain processes similar functions for the left side of the body (Table 6.2).

## Motor and Sensory Areas

Perhaps the easiest areas of the brain to understand and explain are the motor strip and sensory strip (Fig. 6.2). If a surgeon were to take off a person's skull and the coverings of the brain to expose the motor strip of the frontal lobe and introduce a small amount of electrical current (stimulus) on the brain-surface in the finger area (Fig. 6.3, area 1), the awake patient might see some twitching of the index finger of his hand. If this were done to the left side of the brain, the right index finger might twitch. Were the surgeon to move the current slightly up or down the strip, it might cause another finger to move. Moving the current to the face area (2) would cause facial movements; in area 3, the arm on the right side of the body might jerk. These movements are, in a sense, little seizures, a slight seizure induced by the surgeon's electrical stimulus.

If the electrical stimulus comes from within the brain cells themselves (rather than from a surgeon's electrical stimulus), caused for example by a scar, a stroke, or a tumor, the resulting movement would be called a "seizure." If the seizure stays local (focal), it may consist of just the repeated twitch of a finger, a hand, or the face. If the seizure focus is in the sensory strip (Fig. 6.3) and occurs in area 4, then the patient may experience a tingling or funny feeling in the hand (on the opposite side of the body); or if the seizure began at area 5, then the feeling might be in the face or lip.

Focal motor or focal sensory seizures such as these do occur. Trina's seizures (see page 57) are focal motor seizures involving the lip and face, occasionally spreading locally to involve one side of her face. Seizures may start locally, then spread slowly or rapidly to include other areas of the brain. When a focal seizure spreads to other parts of the brain, the initial movement or sensation is the aura, or warning of bigger things to come.

## The Temporal Lobes: Lateral (Outside)

The outside of the left *temporal lobe* is involved in aspects of speech. Someone with a problem in one of these areas may have difficulties in finding the correct word to use; the person may know the correct word and yet be unable to say it, or be able to say words (or repeat words) but not be able to say them clearly, or may be able to talk clearly and

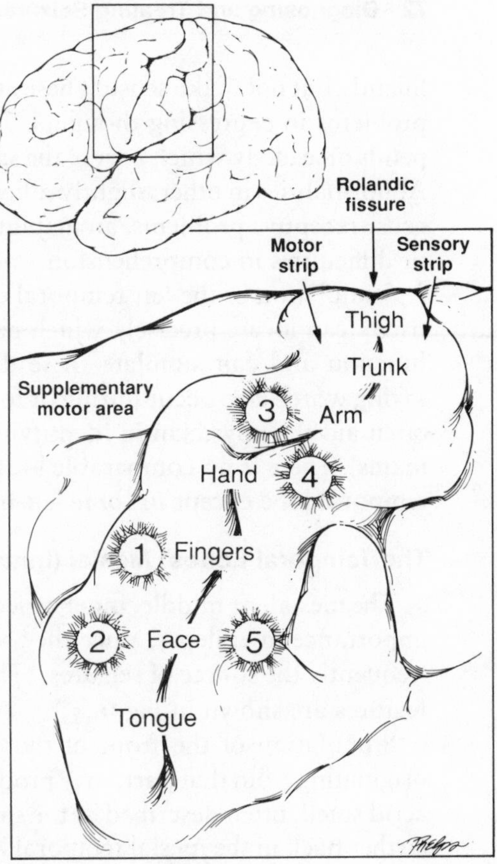

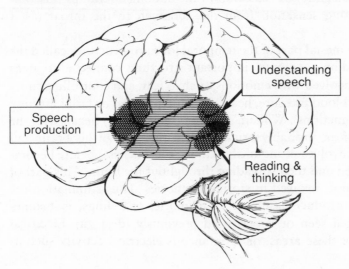

**Figure 6.3.** Motor and sensory areas of the brain. Electrical stimulation at area 1 causes twitching of the finger; at 2, facial movements; at 3, jerking of the arm; at 4 in the sensory strip, tingling in the hand; at 5, tingling of face or lips.

Rolandic fissure

Motor strip

Sensory strip

Thigh

Trunk

Supplementary motor area

Arm

Hand

Fingers

Face

Tongue

**Figure 6.4.** Speech and language areas of the brain. Areas in the temporal (and frontal) lobe, usually on the left side, are responsible for speech and language. Specific functions appear to lie in relatively discrete areas on the outside of the brain.

Understanding speech

Speech production

Reading & thinking

fluently but not make sense. These are all called "expressive" problems, problems in expressing thoughts. The type of expressive problem depends on exactly which part of the speech area is involved (see Fig. 6.4). Abnormalities in other, slightly different areas of the temporal lobe may cause receptive problems, an inability to understand words or phrases, or difficulties in comprehension.

Stimulation of the left temporal cortex with small amounts of electricity can locate precisely which part of the brain is involved in each function and can simulate these difficulties. Problems in finding or saying words also occur during or following focal seizures and thus can often aid the physician in identifying where the seizure begins (or remains). There is no comparable localization on the outside of the right temporal lobe except in *some* left-handed individuals.

### The Temporal Lobes: Mesial (Inner)

The mesial, or middle, inner aspect of both temporal lobes is of great importance in epilepsy, since they are quite prone to damage and are frequently the source of seizures. (This side of the brain and some of its features are shown in Fig. 6.5.)

Stimulation of the front of the mesial temporal lobe, or seizures originating from that part, may produce a smell, usually an unpleasant, acrid smell, often described as the smell of burning rubber. Stimulation farther back in the mesial temporal lobe may produce abnormalities of taste (bitter, metallic) or sensation in the abdomen (cramps, discomfort) or a rising sensation from the abdomen to the throat (as if nauseated).

Also in the mesial part of the temporal lobe are structures called the amygdala and hippocampus, important structures connected to areas of the brain involved with emotions, such as fear, and controlling functions such as blood pressure, heart rate, and paleness or facial flushing (autonomic functions). William's seizure (see page 57) began with the sensation of fear, probably originating in this part of his brain and spreading to involve autonomic functions (the paleness) before becoming generalized and then spreading throughout the brain. This part of the brain is also involved in storing memories. Thus stimulation (or seizures) may produce flashbacks or memories or feelings, as if something had been seen or experienced previously (déjà vu). Electrical stimulation of these areas, or spontaneous electrical activity such as

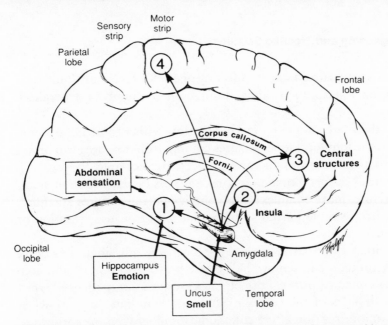

**Figure 6.5.** Temporal lobe, inner side, and spread of seizures. The inner side of the lobe, often involved in seizures. Change in functions during a seizure can indicate the location of the electrical discharge. The amygdala, hippocampus, and uncus are among the most important of these areas. With their many interconnections to the frontal lobe, they influence emotions, consciousness, and autonomic function. If a seizure starts in the uncus, the aura may be an unpleasant smell. It may then spread to the hippocampus (1), followed by a sensation of fear, or to the insula (2), causing abdominal sensation, then spread to other central structures (3), causing loss of awareness and a complex partial seizure, or to the motor area (4), causing a tonic-clonic seizure.

seizures, may create or recreate one, all, or any combination of these feelings and experiences.

Seizures that begin in the temporal lobes may remain focal or may spread slowly or rapidly. For example, seizures starting in the uncus (Fig. 6.5) may initially just consist of a peculiar smell (such as burning rubber). This may be the only thing that happens during a seizure, or the seizure may spread to the hippocampus (1) and be followed by a sensation of fear. The spread may be to the insula (2) and cause a rising sensation in the abdomen and chest or abdominal discomfort. Further spread to area 3 may lead to loss of awareness with staring, often accompanied by automatic, unconsciously repeated movements, such as lip smacking, picking at one's clothes, and wandering around aimless and confused. These movements are called automatisms. Spread of the discharge from the temporal lobe in a different direction (4) may lead to a focal motor seizure, a seizure affecting one side of the body (unilateral seizure), or a seizure spreading throughout the brain (a generalized seizure).

Since there are so many diverse functions either in or closely connected to the temporal lobe, seizures coming from this area can have a variety of manifestations and appearances. For example, the focal seizures (partial seizures) that alter consciousness (a blank look or stare) are, therefore, more complex; thus complex partial seizures are differentiated from simple partial seizures that tend to cause sensation or movement.

Consciousness, or awareness, is not located in any single area of the brain. A surgeon can remove half of the brain (either half) and consciousness remains intact. Loss of consciousness is experienced when either both sides of the cortex dysfunction simultaneously or when there is an interruption of the communication between the cortex and the more centrally located parts of the brain. Alterations in consciousness can be seen naturally during sleep when the electrical activity of the cortex changes. During seizures that involve alterations in consciousness, the electrical activity of the cortex as a whole is always altered.

### The Frontal Lobes

Areas of the frontal lobes other than the motor strip are less well defined; they have to do with personality, memory, anxiety, alertness, and awareness. With many connections to the temporal lobes (Fig. 6.5), it is often difficult to determine from the way the seizure looks whether the function (or the dysfunction of seizures) comes from the frontal or the temporal lobes. Some areas near the "motor strip" (supplementary motor area) (Fig. 6.3) seem to control the coordination of movements of groups of muscles. Electrical stimulation of the supplementary motor area (or seizures) thus may cause the eyes, head, and body to turn away from the side stimulated. Other seizures originating here may appear to cause a brief staring and loss of awareness before some of the stereotyped seizures called complex partial seizures appear.

### Other Areas of the Brain: The Occipital Lobes and Parietal Lobes

The temporal lobes and the frontal lobes are the most important in a discussion of epilepsy because they are most "epileptogenic." We don't know why.

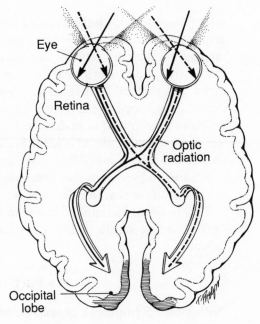

**Figure 6.6.** Occipital lobe, visual pathways. Vision is located in this lobe. An image on a person's right side is seen by the left portion of the retina; electrical impulses from the left side of the retina travel through the visual pathways to the occipital lobe of the cortex on the left side.

Scars, tumors, and other damage in the temporal and frontal lobes of the brain are much more likely to be accompanied by seizures than damage to the occipital lobes or parietal lobes. However, just for completeness, we will briefly discuss these areas as well.

The primary function of the occipital lobe, located in the back of the brain (Fig. 6.6), is vision. Messages from the retina (the back of the eyeball) are transmitted by way of the optic (eye) nerves and by a pathway (the optic radiation) to the occipital lobe, where vision is registered by the brain. Objects off to your left side (when you look straight ahead) are "seen" by the right side of your retina (Fig. 6.6) and proceed along the path to the right side of your brain. Objects on your right (when you look straight ahead) go to the left side of your brain. Vision is complex, and when one stimulates the occipital cortex electrically, the patient sees only bright lights in a random pattern. When a seizure begins in the occipital lobe—which is not common—flashing bright lights may be experienced off to the left side, if it occurs in the right cortex, or to the left side if the right cortex is involved.

The parietal lobe is where "it" all comes together, where much of what we sense by vision or touch achieves meaning. Here, those flashing lights become patterns constituting a formed visual image; through interconnections with the frontal lobe (where memories are stored), we are able to store the images as memories or to recall the formed image as recognized faces or scenes. The posterior temporal-parietal lobe is the site where sounds heard become the pattern of words, which are recognized and remembered or given meaning by association with prior experiences stored in the frontal lobes. It is where speech that is heard becomes speech that is understood and where the sense of touch and feel of a particular object is identified as a key, a ball, or a block. Thus, the parietal lobe is called "the association cortex." It is rarely the source of seizures and seems to play little role in our understanding of the types of epilepsy. It is not, in other words, very "epileptogenic."

This basic and simplified lesson in anatomy should provide a better understanding of the many variations of partial seizures discussed below.

## Simple Partial Seizures

### With Motor Symptoms or with Sensory Symptoms

"Simple partial" seizures may involve movement, with jerking of the foot, face, arm, or any other part of the body. They may involve the senses, with a peculiar tingling, burning, or abnormal sensation in any part of the body. The jerking or sensation will depend on where in the brain the electrical activity begins and how it spreads. Since motor and sensory functions are lateralized—one side of the brain controlling the other side of the body—the motor jerking or sensory feeling will be one-sided, on the side opposite the brain's activity.

Partial seizures may stay local or spread slowly up or down the motor strip or the sensory strip (Fig. 6.1) in a slow spread or "march" that used to be called a "Jacksonian seizure."

### With Autonomic Symptoms

Since a seizure may begin in areas of the brain that control involuntary functions (Fig. 6.5), it may start with the face becoming pale or flushed. The heart may begin to beat rapidly; there may be abdominal cramps and discomfort or a fullness in the chest or throat. Physicians call these "autonomic" symptoms because it is the autonomic part of the nervous system that regulates involuntary body functions like heart rate, blood pressure, and bowel function.

Since the autonomic system has to control both sides of the body simultaneously, not a single half at a time, the physician often cannot identify the side of the origin of the seizure.

## With Psychic Symptoms

Seizures coming from certain parts of the brain can either trigger or stimulate emotions or stimulate the recall of prior experiences. Fear is one emotion frequently experienced alone or as the aura of a seizure, as in William's case. The emotion is often described in vague language: "I just felt scared." "I can't describe it—it's a weird feeling." "I know something's going to happen, I know it's coming." A child may not be able to describe "it" at all, but his face has a frightened look and he comes running to his parent and holds on tightly. But, occasionally, feelings expressed are more specific. A scene experienced in the past will recur to the brain spontaneously; voices will be heard, though often they cannot be understood. (These feelings must be carefully differentiated from the hallucination of drugs or psychiatric illness.) Occasionally a person will have the sensation of déjà vu, that he has experienced something before (even if it has not previously occurred) or that he has seen someone before, or an experience of jamais vu (never seen), when something or someone very familiar seems to be unknown.

Similar experiences may have occurred to each of us on occasion. But when they recur, when they are frequent, or when they are associated with other episodic changes in function or behavior, they may be simple partial seizures.

❑ **Olga comes running to her mother. "I've got that feeling in my hand again. I think I'm going to have another seizure." In a few moments she develops jerking of the arm and then of the whole side of her body. What kind of a seizure is this? Where did it start in the brain? Would it have been a different kind of seizure if it began with jerking in the hand or foot, or with autonomic or psychic symptoms?**

All such events are simple partial seizures starting in different areas of the brain. They may or may not spread to involve other brain areas.

## Complex Partial Seizures

Because the functions located in the temporal lobe and in the frontal lobe are complex (Fig. 6.7), seizures beginning there can be very complex. There are, in addition, many interconnections of both frontal and

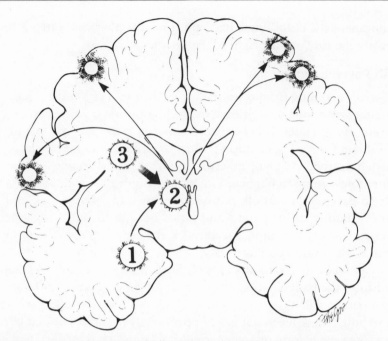

**Figure 6.7.** Spread of partial seizures, simple and complex. If electrical activity remains confined to area 1, there is a simple partial seizure, manifested possibly by sensory, autonomic, or psychic symptoms, all functions located in the temporal lobe. If activity spreads to 2, an area that controls consciousness, alertness, and awareness, cortical function is altered and the patient stares, is confused, or wanders aimlessly in a complex partial seizure with a simple partial onset. If the spread from 1 to 2 is so rapid that symptoms of the seizure in area 1 are not detected *or* if the seizure begins at 3 (in the frontal lobe), and spreads to 2, it will produce the same alterations in consciousness. This is also a complex partial seizure.

temporal lobes to areas of the brain—centrally located—that control alertness and awareness. Thus seizures beginning in the temporal or frontal lobe may alter consciousness. If they do, they are termed "complex partial seizures."

## With Simple Partial Onset

A simple partial seizure may spread quickly to the areas that affect consciousness and result in staring, confusion, loss of alertness, or aimless movements. These are called complex partial seizures "with simple partial onset." They are simple partial seizures with a secondary spread sufficiently slow so that we can recognize where they started. These seizures are most likely to begin in the temporal lobe.

## With Loss of Consciousness at Onset

Complex partial seizures may not produce changes in behavior or function before alterations in consciousness occur. The child may start with a blank stare without any warning or aura, then wander around the room, pick at his clothes, do repetitive movements, and so on. Such seizures, with sudden impairment of consciousness, are likely to originate in the frontal lobe.

Distinguishing between these two types of complex partial seizures—with simple partial onset and with loss of consciousness at onset—may be difficult or impossible. It may require careful analysis of a video-EEG where the instantaneous correlation of changes in the EEG and changes in behavior recorded by the video can be seen. The correct differentiation between these two subtypes is not important unless surgery is being considered.

*Again, before a physician can classify a seizure, she must be sure that a child is actually having seizures. Therefore, diagnosis and classification go hand in hand.*

One of the most confusing areas of classification both for physicians and for parents is differentiation between absence seizures (see page 62) and complex partial seizures. This differentiation may be important since it may determine which medications should be used to treat your child. Further confusion comes when you try to differentiate either of these staring spells from normal daydreaming. Let us give you an example of how we try to differentiate daydreaming from seizures.

❏ **The teacher has called and says Lisa is daydreaming in school. You have noticed some episodes of "daydreaming" at the dinner table. Does she have absence seizures? Does she have atypical absence seizures? Does she have complex partial seizures or is she daydreaming?**

The questions your physician will want to ask you about Lisa are:

• "How frequently is she having these episodes?" Daydreaming would occur infrequently and be situational. Absence seizures may occur many times a day. Complex partial seizures rarely occur more than several times a day or a week.

• "How do these episodes begin?" While most seizures have an abrupt onset, occasionally complex partial seizures begin slowly and a warning precedes them. Daydreaming usually does not start abruptly.

• "Can you interrupt these episodes?" Daydreaming can easily be interrupted by calling Lisa's name or by physically touching her. Seizures, on the other hand, cannot be interrupted.

• "How long does the episode last?" Daydreaming can go on until something else catches a child's attention. Absence seizures rarely last more than fifteen seconds. Complex partial seizures may last up to several minutes.

• "What does the child do during the episode?" While daydreaming or during absence seizures, the child is likely to stare into space. During complex partial seizures, the child is likely to smack her lips, pick at her clothes, or display other automatisms.

• "What is the child like when she 'comes back?'" The child who is daydreaming or having an absence seizure immediately is alert. The child with a complex partial seizure is usually confused for seconds or minutes.

• "Does the child remember what was said during the episode?" While daydreaming, the child may be aware of what is happening but not pay attention. During a seizure, the child is not fully aware of what is happening around her.

• "Do the spells occur only at special times?" If they happen only, say, in math or geography class, the child is likely to be daydreaming. If they occur at random times or whenever the child is tired, they are more likely to be seizures.

With these careful observations, you and your physician can usually differentiate the type of episode.

### With Secondary Generalization

All partial seizures may at times spread to affect the whole brain. While this usually results in a tonic-clonic seizure (see Generalized Seizures above), an atonic seizure in which a child suddenly collapses to the floor or is thrown down, or a tonic seizure in which the child suddenly stiffens and arches his back may result from this spread, depending on the direction of electrical spread.

The parent should carefully observe the onset of a seizure and its progression to enable the physician to take an accurate history in order to determine if there was focal onset, aura, or warning. As with focal or partial seizures, a focal onset of a generalized seizure implies a focal problem or disturbance. Generalized seizures with focal onset require an especially careful medical evaluation, because *if* these seizures cannot be controlled with medication, *and* if the focus can be identified, there may be a possibility of a "cure" of the seizures by surgical removal of the area where the seizure begins.

Now with an understanding of the brain and how it works and with some understanding of its organization and anatomy, you should be better able to understand the many kinds of seizures and the different names physicians use when they describe your child's seizure or seizures. This naming is important because it will help determine the treatment for your child.

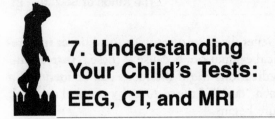

# 7. Understanding Your Child's Tests: EEG, CT, and MRI

The physician's diagnosis of seizures or epilepsy is made *only* by reviewing the history of the episode or by seeing an episode. There is *no* test for epilepsy.

Certain tests, such as the electroencephalogram (EEG) or video-monitoring can be very helpful in determining the type of seizure and in assisting the physician to decide the type of medication to use. Scans of the brain, such as the CT scan or the MRI, can, at times, be useful in localizing an abnormality that may be causing the seizures. Since most children with epilepsy will have these tests on one or more occasions, it is helpful for you as a parent to understand their utility and their limitations. First, the most common of such tests, the EEG.

## The Electroencephalogram (EEG)

We know that the firing of neurons in the brain is carefully modulated by the balance of excitation and inhibition of cells, and that groups of cells work together, interacting by exciting or inhibiting one another. The EEG (electroencephalogram) measures the electricity given off by the brain cells as they interact. The tiny amounts of electricity generated by the brain cells detected on the scalp, if amplified many hundreds of times, can be transformed by the EEG machine and recorded by pens on sheets of graph paper (Fig. 7.1, 7.2).

In most children without epilepsy, EEG recordings resemble wiggly lines, the tiny waves varying slightly in height. In most people *with* epilepsy, abnormalities can be seen on the EEG. These are little bursts of electrical activity, called "sharp waves" or "spikes," that interrupt normal rhythm. These bursts are the result of the electrical discharge of a somewhat larger population of cells all firing simultaneously, actually small, micro-electrical seizures within very tiny areas of the brain. They are not clinically detectable seizures because the spikes and sharp waves do not represent *enough* cells firing simultaneously to "alter the function or behavior" of the person.

If your child already has had a seizure, he probably has also had an EEG. It doesn't hurt and it shouldn't, therefore, be frightening. If your child has not had an EEG, he should be told what to expect. The explanation should, of course, be tailored to the child's age and level of understanding. Going to a strange place is frightening, so is separation from parents. And having "gook" put in your hair and wires on your head can be alarming. If the child knows exactly what will happen and why, he will be reassured, even intrigued, by the procedure. So will you.

The EEG technician who performs the test usually has had special training in working with children. He or she will explain that because the wires are to be put in special places the child's head will be measured. The wires will be stuck to the scalp either with a form of clay or paste or with collodion, a mixture that smells and acts like airplane glue. This procedure often will be done with the young child sitting in the mother's lap or, with the older child or adult, sitting in a chair or lying on a padded table (Fig. 7.3). *There is no pain or discomfort.* Many children report that the worst part of the test is getting the "junk" out of their hair afterward!

Because the EEG is best done when a person is relaxed, the room will be quiet and darkened. EEGs should be done when a child is awake (but quiet) and also when he is asleep because some abnormalities show up in one state but not in the other. Many EEG laboratories give the child medicine so he will go to sleep, and older children and adults often fall asleep spontaneously in the relaxing atmosphere of the EEG lab during the hour, approximately, the test usually takes. In special circumstances the EEG may last a longer or a shorter time, depending on what information the physician needs.

Usually you may stay with your child to provide reassurance, but only if you also are quiet and still. Any movement and any touching or patting your child may cause electrical disturbances that show up on this very sensitive machine and confuse the EEG tracing. A child's muscle movements—crying, squirming, squeezing the eyes shut, or

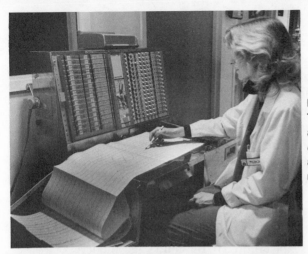

**Figure 7.1.** The EEG machine. The technician carefully follows and makes notes about the EEG, *e.g.,* whether the child is awake, asleep, moving, and how he is responding.

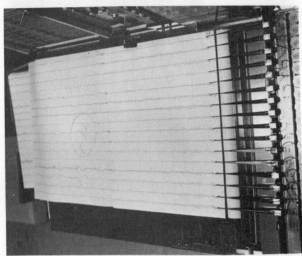

**Figure 7.2.** Normal resting EEG. Note normal rhythms, like ripples on a lake. Each line (channel) made by a pen represents a different area of the brain.

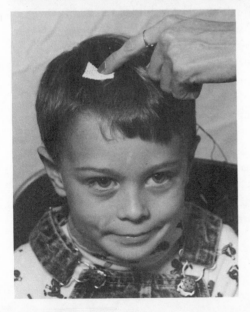

**Figure 7.3.** The electroencephalogram (EEG). After an area of the scalp is cleaned off by a technician the electrode is put in place with a paste-like substance.

clenching the teeth—can cause the EEG machine to go "crazy" as it picks up the electricity from the muscles. Relaxation and quiet for parent and child both are crucial to a good recording.

• Yes, your child may eat before the test.

• Yes, your child should sleep normally the night before a test unless, as on a rare occasion, your physician wants a "sleep-deprived" EEG.

• Yes, your child may bring a favorite doll, soft toy, or blanket if that will make him more comfortable.

## Normalities and Abnormalities on the EEG

Most of the pen movements on the EEG are common and normal (Fig. 7.4A–D).

When muscles twitch or contract, they produce electricity, and this electricity is picked up on the EEG. When people blink their eyes ("eye movement artifact"), this movement also is seen on the EEG. Artifact means that it is not coming from the brain, so it doesn't count. ("Eye movement artifact" is shown in Fig. 7.5A.) Muscle "artifacts" can be seen when the child clenches his teeth (Fig. 7.5B). Even during the process of falling asleep, changes are produced in the rhythm of the EEG that look like bursts of abnormal electrical activity (Fig. 7.4D). None of these changes in rate or rhythm on the EEG are abnormal, so don't worry.

Only three abnormalities on the EEG are of importance in the diagnosis and management of seizures: spikes, slowing, and evidence of seizures. Each of these may be either focal (local), or generalized. Each has a different meaning.

REMEMBER: A seizure is an electrical discharge from the brain which causes a change (alteration) in movement or behavior. If there is *no* change in behavior or movement, this is not a *clinical* seizure. Some abnormalities on the EEG may be called *electrical* seizures, but electrical seizures are rarely treated.

The EEG may:

• Show electrical changes that indicate either an electrical abnormality in one area of the brain or electrical abnormalities in many areas of the brain;

• Indicate to your physician that there is a specific area of the brain of concern;

**Figure 7.4.** EEG of normal infant and teenager. The record (A) shows an awake infant blinking (closed arrow) and muscle artifact (open arrow), both in the first line or channel. Much normal slowing is seen throughout the record. (B) The bottom two lines or channels show the rhythmical fast activity of the infant asleep, called spindles; the two upper channels show a normal amount of slow activity that resembles in many respects the awake record. In the EEG of an awake teenager (C), when the eyes close (arrow), very rhythmical activity, known as the basic rhythm, appears in the bottom line; (D) sleep recording in the same teenager with a K complex (arrow) seen normally in sleep.

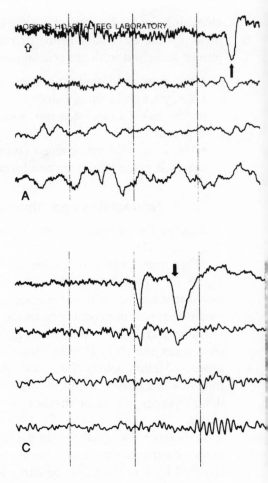

• Help your physician to determine the type of seizure your child had;

• Indicate which medication is most likely to be most effective for controlling that type of seizure.

Diagnosis of seizures or epilepsy depends on an accurate interpretation of the events that have occurred. The diagnosis of a seizure or of epilepsy is *not* made by the EEG alone. Furthermore, an EEG does not diagnose or rule out epilepsy. Some people with abnormal EEGs never have seizures. Some people with seizures have normal EEGs.

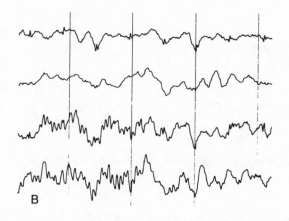

B

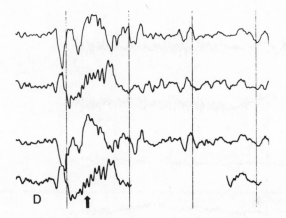

D

## Spikes

Since a clinical seizure requires that a sufficient number of brain cells fire together to cause the alteration in movement or behavior, one would expect this "firing" to cause a change in the electrical activity recorded on the EEG. That is exactly what does happen. The normal EEG (Fig. 7.4C) represents an almost random firing of brain cells; when the cells fire simultaneously they produce an electrical abnormality in the EEG called a "spike" (Fig. 7.6A).

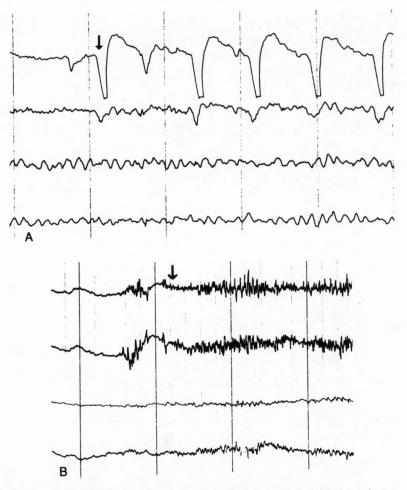

**Figure 7.5.** Normal EEG with eye movement and muscle artifacts. With the patient blinking (A), the EEG (arrow) record shows the movement of the eyes. In B, the arrow shows muscle activity when the patient bites down or chews.

A spike is a mini-*electrical* seizure. Only if that electrical disturbance spreads to involve more cells (a sufficient number to change behavior) would a true *clinical* seizure occur. Thus, repeated spikes coming from a particular area represent the local response to a provocation there, an epileptic focus or scar. In a child (or adult) who has had a focal seizure, spikes may indicate the area of the brain where the seizure started (Fig. 7.6A).

Multifocal spikes (Fig. 7.6B), by comparison, suggest that there are many abnormal areas of the brain.

Spikes are not of significance unless they are found consistently in one area.

### Slowing

The rhythm of the normal EEG varies with the child's age and differs depending on whether the child is awake, drowsy, or asleep. There are well-established limits for these normal variations in rate and rhythm. Slowing may be either focal (Fig. 7.6C) or generalized (Fig. 7.6D).

A common cause of slowing is post-ictal, occurring after a seizure, due to "inhibition" of the firing of cells. It may last several hours. Post-ictal slowing is best diagnosed by its disappearance soon after the seizure. If slowing lasts for days after a seizure, further evaluation is necessary.

*Focal slowing should always be of concern and requires careful evaluation because it may occur in association with a local disturbance of the brain, such as a concussion, a stroke, or a tumor. In a child who has had a seizure, focal slowing on an EEG (unlike focal spikes) may, therefore, require further studies and appropriate treatment.*

Slowing all over the brain—generalized slowing—signifies disturbed brain function caused by acute disturbances of whole brain function—for example, chemical disturbances, lack of oxygen, infection, or severe head injury with loss of consciousness. Generalized slowing may also be seen in children with long-standing chronic brain dysfunction.

## EEG Abnormalities Related to Certain Seizure Types

While the EEG does not diagnose seizures, certain abnormalities on the EEG are commonly associated with certain seizure types and can help your physician determine your child's treatment and the probable outcome. Thus, just as classification of seizures is useful, so classification of the EEG is useful also.

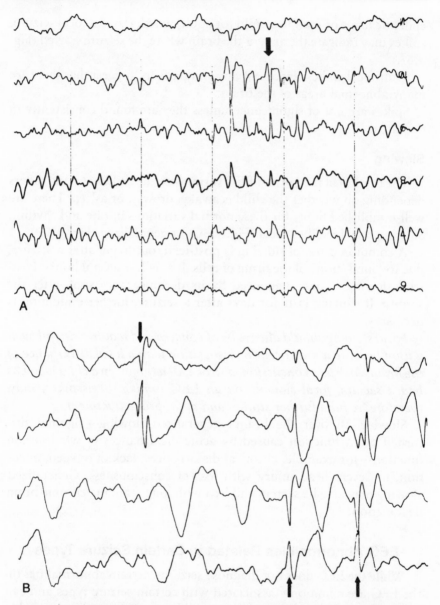

**Figure 7.6.** Abnormal EEGs. Each channel (line) on the EEG represents a different area of the brain. In A, the pointed spikes (arrow) come from the part of the brain under the electrodes measured by channels 2 and 3, showing that the abnormality is partial (focal) in that specific area of the brain. In B, the multi-focal spikes (arrows) appear in several channels, showing that they arise in several different areas of the brain and that there are multi-focal abnormalities of the underlying brain. In C, the top three channels

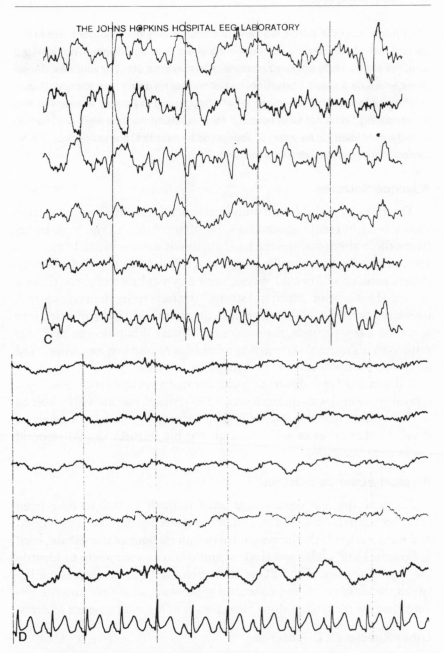

THE JOHNS HOPKINS HOSPITAL EEG LABORATORY

from the left side of the head show high amplitude with slow waves, as compared to electrical activity from the right side of the head (bottom three lines). In D, all channels show low-voltage slow activity, as might be seen in a child in a coma.

❏ **Roger is in the third grade and has been a very good student. But in the second half of the year the teacher sends you a note that Roger is not working up to his ability. He is not paying attention in class; he often daydreams. Sometimes, when he's asked a question, he claims that he didn't hear the question or that he has forgotten the answer. What's happening to Roger? Is he bored and daydreaming? Is he not smart enough to understand the new work and, consequently, confused? Is he upset or depressed by events at home or school? Is he having staring spells (absence seizures)?**

## Absence Seizures

The EEG in a child with simple absence (petit mal) seizures often shows brief bursts of spike and wave abnormalities (Fig. 7.7). In between these abnormalities the basic rhythm is quite normal. Sometimes spontaneously, but usually with hyperventilation, the EEG demonstrates runs of spikes and waves, with a typical rate of three times a second. This type of "electrical storm," if it lasts more than one second, interferes with the child's alertness or awareness. He will stare into space for a few seconds, then may say, "What? What did you say?" He returns to his normal state just as quickly as he had lost awareness. The EEG also abruptly returns to normal background.

If Roger has typical staring spells during hyperventilation and has a typical spike and wave pattern on his EEG, the physician will be able to tell his mother that these spells will be outgrown, that he is unlikely to develop other types of seizures, and that his seizures should respond easily to medication.

## Atypical Absence Seizures

Atypical absence seizures are often difficult to differentiate from complex partial seizures. The number of spells per day, the age of onset, and most particularly the associated manifestations of the seizure, such as lip smacking, picking at clothes, and confusion may help to identify the type of seizure. The EEG is also often useful in distinguishing between the classical three-per-second spike-wave of simple absence seizures and the somewhat slower spike-wave of atypical absence seizures.

## Other Special EEG Patterns

"Hypsarrhythmia," a very chaotic, high-voltage EEG pattern (Fig. 7.8) of spikes, poly-spikes, and slow waves seen in some young children of six months to three years, is almost always associated with the severe

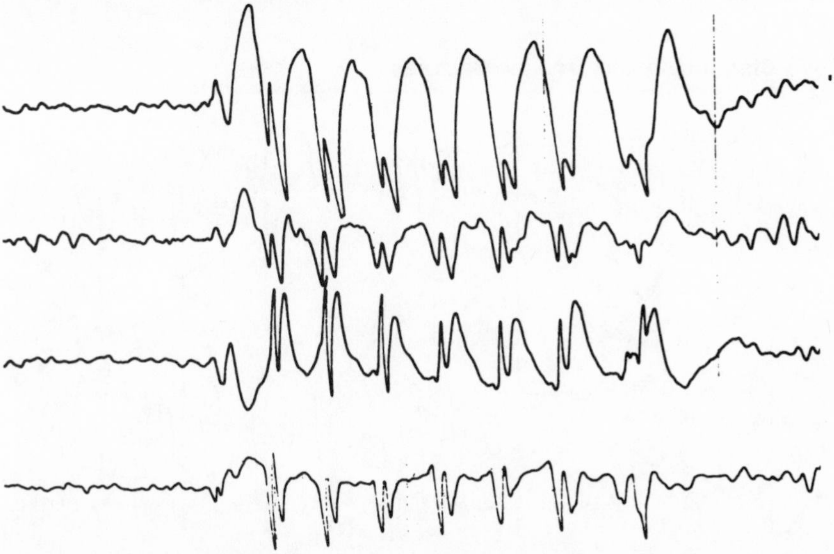

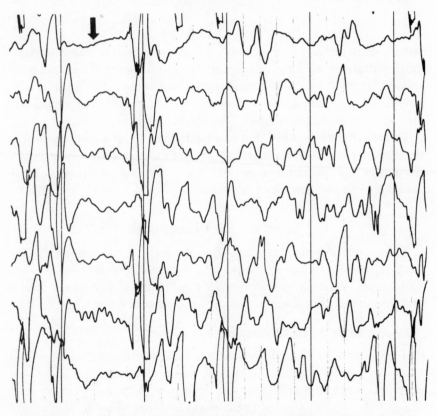

**Figure 7.7.** Spike-wave abnormality. These brief bursts of spike-wave activity, preceded and followed by normal activity, are often associated with absence seizures.

**Figure 7.8.** Hypsarrhythmic EEG. Chaotic, high-amplitude EEG with multi-focal spikes, with a brief voltage suppression (arrow), usually seen in association with infantile spasms.

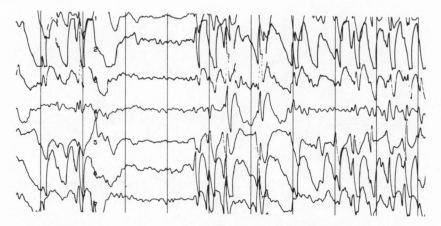

**Figure 7.9.** The Lennox-Gastaut pattern. Bursts of high amplitude spikes and slow waves are less regular and well-organized than the spike-wave activity of absence seizures.

seizure disorder infantile spasms (see Chapter 8). The "Lennox-Gastaut" pattern is also a chaotic pattern of slow spike-wave and polyspikes (Fig. 7.9), a pattern seen in some children and young adults who have a mixed seizure disorder. The term is used to describe the EEG and also the seizure syndrome (see Chapter 8).

Other types of epilepsy that can be diagnosed by a combination of the clinical pattern of the seizures and the EEG include benign rolandic seizures, which have midtemporal or parietal spikes, and juvenile myoclonic epilepsy of Janz (see Chapter 8).

## Special EEG Procedures

Three special procedures that may be part of the routine EEG—sleep-induction, hyperventilation, and photic stimulation—are called "activation" procedures because they can "activate" patterns of abnormalities on the EEG. Such procedures should be routine with children.

### "Why do they do the test both awake and asleep?"

The EEG looks quite different, depending on whether the patient is awake or asleep (Fig. 7.10A and B). Some abnormalities, spikes for example, may be apparent only in a drowsy or sleep state because sleep changes the organization of brain waves and may allow hidden abnor-

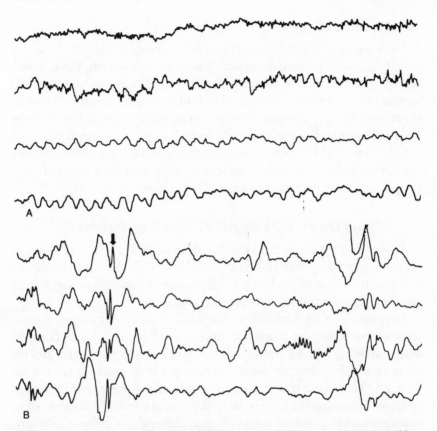

**Figure 7.10.** (A) Normal awake EEG of three-year-old. (B) The same three-year-old asleep shows spike activity (arrow).

malities to show up. Some children with epilepsy may have a normal EEG awake and a very abnormal EEG when asleep.

### *"What is hyperventilation, and why is it done?"*

The technician will ask your child to breathe deeply, thus causing changes in the blood carbon dioxide and usually resulting in slowing on the EEG. Such changes as a consequence of hyperventilating are far more pronounced in younger children than in older ones. They can reveal abnormalities on the EEG. In children with absence seizures, overbreathing can even cause a clinical spell and allow the EEG characteristics of this form of epilepsy to become overt.

### *"What is photic stimulation?"*

Flashing lights also may trigger seizures. A special class of seizures is called "photic sensitive seizures." Using a stroboscopic light, which flashes at frequencies from one per second to sixty per second, the EEG technician can observe whether the child is "photic sensitive," that is, that the child's EEG responds to certain frequencies of flashes, with the EEG showing spikes every time the light flashes. Occasionally, "photic driving" can make the brain so active that a real seizure will occur, one similar to episodes that occur under nonlaboratory conditions in a few people, who are then said to have "photic sensitive epilepsy."

## "Why Do an EEG Anyway? And Why Repeat It?"

"I still don't understand why one does an EEG," you say. "You've said it doesn't diagnose epilepsy. You've stated that it doesn't rule out epilepsy. It sounds to me like it's useless, one of those boondoggle tests doctors request in order to make more money."

Despite all of its limitations, the EEG *is* useful for comparison if seizures continue, get worse, or change in character. An EEG might detect slowing, thereby possibly suggesting a need for concern, and for other types of testing, or focal spikes, a possible local source for the seizure. The EEG can be helpful in diagnosing some special forms of epilepsy. Therefore the EEG is, indeed, a useful test in the diagnosis and management of children with epilepsy, although, of course, only one part of that diagnosis and management.

"If that's all they get out of the test, why would they want another one?" you might ask. Others might question, "Will the follow-up EEG really show that the epilepsy is getting better or worse?" The answer to both of these questions is that *an EEG should be repeated only when it will provide useful information.* It should not be repeated routinely, say, every three months, every six months, or even every year, since if your child's seizures are controlled, you shouldn't care if the EEG is normal or not, that is, until you want to consider stopping medication.

An EEG should be repeated only if:

• Seizures are continuing despite appropriate medication, or
• Seizures are changing in pattern or frequency, or
• Seizures that have been well controlled now recur, or
• If the child's functioning is changing.

In any of these above circumstances, a change in the EEG could provide a clue to the reason for the change. A person who has had a few generalized tonic-clonic seizures, followed by successful control of seizures, might have only an initial EEG and no further EEG *unless* the physician considers stopping medication, and then a second EEG may provide important information about the possibility of further seizures. A child who has frequent seizures or focal seizures might by way of comparison require many EEGs to determine where the seizures are coming from. A third child with difficult-to-control seizures might also require many EEGs, or even continuous monitoring of the EEG for days, in order to capture the seizures as they occur and identify their origin in order to plan surgery. But continuous EEG monitoring, either with ambulatory (walking around) equipment or video monitoring, is a special test and should be used only in such special circumstances.

So the answer to the question "Why repeat the EEG?" is that it depends. But if your physician wants a repeat, don't hesitate to ask why. He should be able and willing to tell you.

## Intensive EEG Monitoring

For the evaluation of most individuals with epilepsy, no special EEG tests are required. For most such children, the neurological evaluation, an EEG, and in some cases a CT scan or an MRI scan will provide sufficient evaluation. However, in three situations special EEG tests are indicated. The situations are:

• When the individual is having episodes that are not, clearly, seizures; when described to your physician, they do not seem to him to fit any particular seizure type. He will be concerned that these are not true seizures, but rather are pseudo-seizures.
• Special testing is *always* required when surgery is even considered as a possibility. The testing may indicate that the seizures are coming from several different areas of the brain, thus making surgery less likely to be effective. Alternatively, intensive monitoring may indicate that there is sufficient evidence of a focal source for the seizures that it may be worth initiating a series of events and tests which would help in making intelligent decisions about surgery (see Chapter 13).
• Some children with uncontrolled seizures may benefit from

intensive monitoring that might identify the type of seizure and indicate alternative medications.

## Ambulatory EEG Monitoring

Ambulatory monitoring is usually performed with a small tape cassette worn on the belt and attached by small wires to EEG electrodes pasted to the scalp. These cassettes can record EEG for twenty-four hours without a change in the tape. When the person wearing the monitor has an "episode," or feels the warning of an episode, he can push a button; a mark will then be made on the cassette tape. For children it is important to have an observer record the time on the machine and also any suspected or unusual behaviors, data to be correlated later with any abnormalities appearing on the recorded EEG (see Fig. 7.11A, B).

Reading twenty-four hours worth of EEG paper would be cumbersome and time-consuming, but the tapes can be played at sixty times the normal speed with the technician or doctor *listening* for the characteristic sounds of seizures. If such abnormalities are heard, the tape is slowed down and the EEG tracings displayed on a videoscreen for further analysis. This then becomes an efficient method of screening for EEG abnormalities and seizures.

While ambulatory monitoring permits recognition of major brain wave abnormalities, such as generalized spike-wave seizures, it is not, however, precise enough for pre-surgical evaluations. There are also a few additional drawbacks and limitations to the ambulatory monitoring test. Because the child being monitored is usually at home, and because it is not uncommon for one or more of the electrodes to become loose or unglued without anyone knowing, the monitoring may yield less than accurate reports. It may be impossible to interpret any episodes that occur if not all of the electrodes are working. True to Murphy's Law, it is invariably the critical electrode that malfunctions.

It may be difficult to tell what is a seizure and what isn't. If the tape is scanned rapidly, brief events may be missed unless they have been identified earlier by the child or the observer. That is why it is so important for an accurate diary to be maintained during the recording. Also, if events are occurring infrequently, they may not occur at all while the child is being monitored. Thus, ambulatory monitoring is impractical for assessing rare events. Ambulatory monitoring is not for everyone; in selected cases, however, it can be useful.

**Figure 7.11.** (A) Ambulatory EEG monitoring. A child goes about normal activities with EEG recorded on a cassette in the machine carried on the shoulder. (B) The portable cassette recorder and wires sit on the top of the terminal used to read the EEG once it is recorded on a cassette tape. The EEG is then re-formatted by the computer and displayed on screen at left.

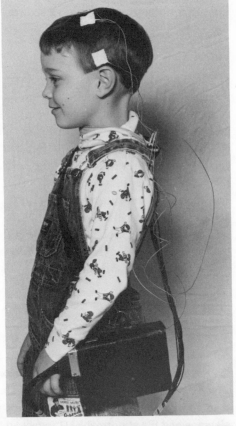

B 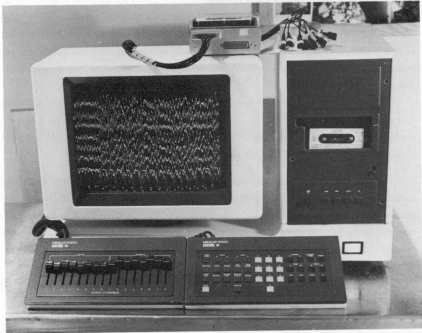 A

## Video-EEG Monitoring

The optimal approach to analysis of seizures is to both see and record their onset and their spread. Such an approach is mandatory in situations in which surgery is being considered. When surgery is even an option, it is critical to know the exact area of the brain involved in the origin of the seizures. Video-EEG monitoring allows recording of the EEG from multiple areas of the brain and also simultaneous video recording of the seizures.

Video-EEG monitoring can also be useful when there is a question about what the spells really are. The ability to see a spell that is said to be a seizure *and* to record the EEG at the same time is the definitive way to differentiate seizures from pseudo-seizures.

Two examples will illustrate:

❑ **Sasha was a fifteen-year-old with a severe behavior disorder and seizures. Despite several years of intensive outpatient psychotherapy, he was once again thrown out of school. His family was exasperated. It was clear to both his neurologist and psychiatrist that he used his seizures to manipulate his environment. He was taken off medication and these peculiar episodes, which did not sound like seizures, did not increase in frequency. The family was taught to ignore them and Sasha seemed able to control them. But their persistence and his abnormal EEG remained of concern to his psychiatrist.**

**The only resolution to his problem was to send him to a residential institution where he could be taught better behavioral control. Since the psychiatrist at the institution was uncomfortable dealing with a child with seizures, we brought him into the monitoring unit to see whether all of his spells were pseudo-seizures.**

**Much to our surprise, while most of his episodes were, indeed, pseudo-seizures, at night he had genuine tonic-clonic seizures. Placing him back on medication eliminated these true seizures and allowed the psychiatrist at the institution to concentrate on his behavioral problems.**

❑ **Simon's seizures began when he was two. They would start in his left foot and spread up the left side. At times, he would have a weakness in the left leg that was thought to be post-ictal paralysis, but at other times the leg was quite normal. Despite intensive attempts with medication, seizures continued to occur several times each day. The EEG showed a focus near the motor strip on the right, and we faced the choice of operating to remove the focus (with the probability of causing paralysis at least of the leg) or of allowing him to continue to**

**have seizures. We decided to wait. After several years, video-EEG monitoring allowed us to see the start of several seizures. The seizures actually began anteriorly in the frontal lobe and then spread into the motor strip. They began in an area that could possibly be removed without damaging his motor ability. Simon was, therefore, put on the list for evaluation with the grid (see Chapter 13) electrodes placed on the surface of his brain and eventually had successful surgery—without experiencing paralysis.**

Intensive monitoring allows us to make decisions we were never able to make before. It gives us the opportunity to separate true seizures definitively from pseudo-seizures and more successfully to identify children as prospects for surgery.

A small, but growing, number of epilepsy centers are now capable of intensive video-EEG monitoring. Video-EEG monitoring is usually carried out in special hospital settings with the patient in bed or sitting in a chair where the video camera and EEG machine can constantly monitor his activities. The EEG and the video are recorded simultaneously (Fig 7.12) in one of several ways which will permit simultaneous analysis of the behavior and the electrical activity. Often these intensive monitoring centers will withdraw medication to precipitate seizures, which can then be recorded.

The principal drawback to this monitoring is its present expense. It requires the use of hospital space and the time of nurses or technicians who will monitor the patient and the equipment twenty-four hours a day. Also, analysis of the records is expensive and time consuming (Fig. 7.13). Because seizures must be of sufficient frequency to make their recording feasible, intensive video-EEG monitoring may require many days in the special monitoring unit at enormous cost. Also, there is far more demand for available monitoring than there is space available, and waiting lists often extend for many months.

However, when seizures are sufficiently frequent and disabling to the individual, or when the localization of the onset of seizures is sufficiently important to future decision-making about the use of the proper medication or the use of surgery, then intensive monitoring, expensive as it is, is cost-effective and worth waiting for. The goals of hospital admission and monitoring must, of course, be carefully defined in advance in order to make the most efficient use of this complex system.

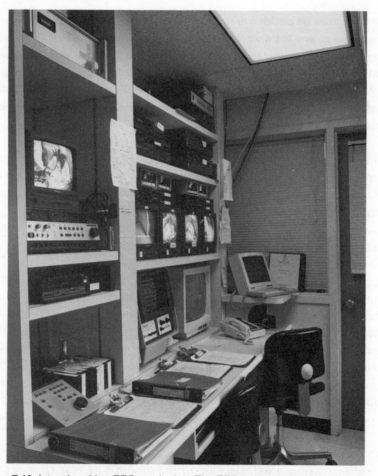

**Figure 7.12.** Intensive video-EEG monitoring. The EEGs of several patients are constantly monitored by the nurses' station. When a seizure occurs, the video and the EEG are stored electronically and can be reviewed later by physicians.

## CT and MRI Scanning

When a child has had a seizure or multiple seizures, the first question parents and physicians ask is, "Why did the seizure occur?" Although more than 50 percent of seizures in children are "idiopathic" (having no known cause) and although most that are "symptomatic" (due to disturbance in the brain) are secondary to something that happened long ago, there is an almost irresistible urge among physicians and families to "take a look," to see if "we can find out why this occurred." Neurologists and neurosurgeons who see adults who have just begun to have seizures often, properly consider brain tumors or vascular (blood vessel) problems as a possible cause of these seizures. The causes of seizures in children are different. Tumors and vascular problems are a rare cause of new onset seizures in children (see Chapter 3).

Modern radiology, through the use of brain scanning, has, fortunately, made it possible to "take a look" relatively easily and at modest expense and without harm to the patient (see table 7.1).

*It is not necessary to do a scan on every child who has had a first seizure.*

There are good reasons for a physician to request a scan if:

• There are focal seizures, or
• There is focal slowing on the EEG, or
• You or your physician are concerned that your child is getting worse.

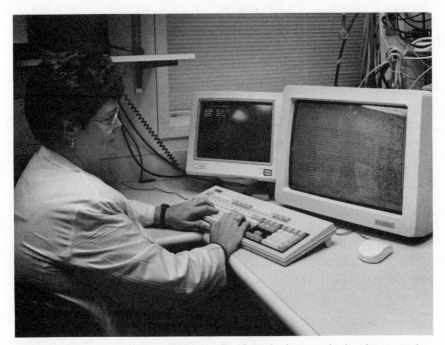

**Figure 7.13.** Analysis of video-EEG data. Dr. Vining is shown reviewing data; note the seizure displayed on the computer screen.

**Table 7.1    Advantages and Disadvantages of Computed Tomographic (CT) and Magnetic Resonance Imaging (MRI) Scans**

| Characteristic | CT scan | MRI scan |
|---|---|---|
| Speed | 10–15 minutes | 45 minutes |
| Ease | Simple, even with sick individuals on life support machines | Difficult with sick patients |
| | Good for screening for calcium | Better for small or subtle changes or problems occurring near bone |
| Cost | Expensive | Very expensive |

But remember that:

• Most scans are normal in children with epilepsy;
• Most abnormalities found will *not* explain the epilepsy;
• Most abnormalities found will *not* lead to a different approach to treatment.

Something abnormal on a scan has not necessarily caused the seizures and may not cause seizures in the future. Only if the abnormality on the scan appears in the proper location of the brain to have caused the seizures can we presume cause and effect.

## CT Scanning

Computerized Tomography (CAT or CT) scanning, a procedure introduced in the early 1970s, has revolutionized the ability to "see" the brain. Low-dose x-rays are detected and interpreted by a computer, which then generates a picture "just as if we had cut a slice of the brain."

The principal reason for a CT scan is to see whether the seizure had a cause that can be treated surgically. The CT can also reveal other causes for which there may be specific treatments.

## MRI Scanning

While CT scanning has revolutionized our ability to see the brain, magnetic resonance imaging (MRI), which is even newer, has increased our ability to see the brain even more clearly. Unlike CT scanning, MRI does not employ x-rays but rather uses a huge magnet to create an image which is then analyzed by computer in a fashion similar to the CT. It produces pictures of even greater detail. The advantages and disadvantages of CT and MRI are shown in Table 7.1.

The principal disadvantages of the MRI are that, with current equipment, a scan takes about forty-five minutes, during which the child must lie perfectly still in the tunnel-like machine and thus may require sedation, and also that the test is more expensive than CT. However, when detail of the brain is important, or when subtle changes must be seen, the MRI is indicated. It produces far better pictures of the brain and of most abnormalities than the CT scan does.

If your physician wants your child to have an EEG or a CT or MRI scan, you should feel free to ask him why he wants the test and what he hopes to learn from it. These questions are even more appropriate if he wants to repeat the test.

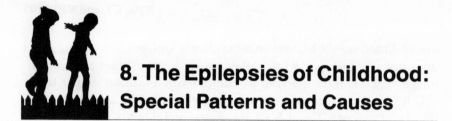

# 8. The Epilepsies of Childhood: Special Patterns and Causes

## Epilepsy and Its Special Forms

Epilepsy is defined as two or more seizures that are not provoked and are not due to an acute disturbance of the brain. Because there are many different types of seizures, epilepsy can take many different forms. There is not, thus, one "epilepsy" but many. Therefore, if we were to speak properly, we would not speak about "epilepsy," but about "the epilepsies or epileptic syndromes."

## Epilepsy Syndromes

In addition to the many types of seizures, there are various patterns of recurrent seizures sufficiently distinctive in their course and outcome and in their response to specific medications to warrant distinct names and separate discussions.

### Benign Rolandic Epilepsy

Benign rolandic epilepsy is a special form of seizures in children. Often starting after three years of age, it has rather typical clinical manifestations and a typical EEG. It is usually "benign" in that it is outgrown at adolescence whether or not it is treated and in that the children are usually normal before, during, and after this form of epilepsy that is outgrown. In many or most cases, the seizures are infrequent and do not need medication.

Seizures in this form of epilepsy usually start with a sensation at the corner of the mouth, followed by jerking of that corner. The jerking may spread to one side of the face or cause a twisting of that side. The seizure may, on occasion, spread throughout that side of the body or become a generalized tonic-clonic seizure. These seizures occur more commonly at night and during certain stages of sleep.

The diagnosis of benign rolandic epilepsy is confirmed by an EEG pattern of repetitive spike activity firing predominantly from the mid-temporal or parietal areas of the brain near the rolandic (motor) strip—hence, the name rolandic epilepsy. Bilateral spike activity on the EEG is not uncommon and inter-ictal activity is more common on the EEG during certain stages of sleep.

The seizures are often so infrequent and benign, occurring only at night, that most children with benign rolandic epilepsy are not treated with medication. If a child's seizures are more frequent or troublesome, carbamazepine can be very effective and may be tapered and discontinued after puberty.

There may be a genetic predisposition to this form of epilepsy.

## Juvenile Myoclonic Epilepsy of Janz

Juvenile myoclonic epilepsy is a relatively newly recognized syndrome unfamiliar to many physicians who do not work in the field of epilepsy. It is easily recognized, if you know what to look for and know what questions to ask of the patient. It is also easily treated.

Epilepsy of Janz starts in late childhood or adolescence, often about the time of puberty. Its hallmark is mild myoclonic jerks, most common as the person is going to sleep or awakening in the morning. An adolescent will describe jerking of the arms or legs, a feeling of being very "jumpy." Some patients have told us that they set their alarm clocks to wake up early and then stay in bed for one half hour to an hour, until the jumpiness wears off. They say that if they get up more quickly the jerking gets much worse.

If a person has early morning seizures, informing your doctor about the jerks that precede them may make it easier to diagnosis this particular form of epilepsy.

Occasionally, the jerking builds up and becomes sufficiently severe so that the person experiences a clonic or a tonic-clonic seizure. In addition, people may experience absence seizures.

The EEG between seizures, in this form of epilepsy, often shows a fast, multiple- or double-spike pattern followed by slow waves, with fast rapid spikes occurring during the jerks. When the diagnosis is suspected, the best way of confirming it is a sleep EEG, continued for ten or fifteen minutes after the person awakens. It is during this time that the jerks and the characteristic EEG pattern are most likely to be seen.

Diagnosis is important because although this form of epilepsy responds poorly to many medications, it is usually easily controlled with valproic acid. The seizures often recur when this medication is withdrawn. A family history of epilepsy may occur in as many as 40 percent of siblings of those with the epilepsy of Janz. Studies of these families are beginning to provide clues to its genetic basis.

### Infantile Spasms

Infantile spasms are a special form of epilepsy of infancy readily recognized clinically, but initially mistaken for colic. In a typical infantile spasm, the child will suddenly flex his head or his body at the waist. The arms come up in a startle-like reaction, the knees are drawn up, and the child may let out a short cry. This spasm lasts just a second or two, then the child relaxes, but the spasm quickly recurs in the same form. These spasms continue in a series of five to fifty or more before the series stops. The child may have many series per day.

Since the mother often thinks that the cry and the flexion represent cramps or pain, her description may sound to the physician as if the child has colic, but *colic does not occur in a series of episodes.*

*Infantile spasms is the only type of epilepsy where seizures occur in series.*

The series of infantile spasms is most likely to occur when the child is drowsy, either waking from a nap or going to sleep. A parent might notice them particularly when the child has been placed in a high-chair for a meal.

Less frequently, the spasms may be extensor, with the head thrown back and the body briefly stiffening while the legs are extended; or the spasm may be unilateral, with one arm coming up, the head turned to that side and the leg on the same side extended. These brief atypical spells also occur in series.

Infantile spasms rarely start before two months of age, and most commonly between four and eight months. Spells that occur in series in this age group are usually infantile spasms or one of its variants. Even untreated, this form of epilepsy gradually disappears during the second to the fourth year of life. However, the child is usually severely handicapped otherwise. Shortly after the spasms begin, these children seem to stop making developmental progress and often lose skills they had previously acquired. A child who had started to sit may stop sitting, may even lose the ability to roll over, may stop babbling, and may function like a much younger child. Because of this deterioration, children with infantile spasms are often thought to have an underlying degeneration of the brain. Only 10 to 20 percent of children with infantile spasms will have normal mental function; the vast majority will have moderate to severe mental retardation. This is the *only* seizure type where one can predict such a poor outlook (prognosis). The poor prognosis is in part a consequence of the underlying brain pathology, but also may in some way be a result of the effects of this chaotic electrical activity in the brain. Some people think that the earlier the treatment of these seizures is initiated, the better the outlook. But even infants whose spasms are brought under control with treatment often develop another special form of epilepsy called the Lennox-Gastaut syndrome.

Infantile spasms may occur in the young child who has developmental problems of the brain or with brain damage caused by birth injury, meningitis, or head trauma. Abnormalities of metabolism such as low blood sugar or amino acid problems may also be responsible. All of these are designated as "symptomatic" infantile spasms, since they are caused by the underlying process. A second and smaller group of infantile spasms are called "cryptogenic" since their cause is unknown. Children with cryptogenic infantile spasms appear perfectly normal in development before the seizures begin.

Infantile spasms are virtually always accompanied by an abnormality of the EEG known as "hypsarrhythmia," a wildly chaotic pattern with multiple spikes and slow waves (see page 93). While it may or may not be true, it is useful to think of this EEG pattern as imposing severe "static" on the brain waves so that the brain functions poorly and the child's functioning deteriorates.

A physician evaluating a child with infantile spasms should search for treatable metabolic causes of the spasms and infectious processes. An EEG and a CT or MRI scan should also be requested. Unless a specific treatable condition is found, and one rarely is, treatment for the spasms should begin promptly.

We initially treat all such children with ACTH (adrenocorticotropic hormone), a form of steroid given twice a day by intramuscular injection. However, some physicians use oral steroids, benzodiazepines such as diazepam (Valium) or clonazepam (Klonopin), or valproic acid (Depakote, Depakene). The relative effectiveness of these various forms of treatment has not been tested, nor has the duration of treatment been established. Each treatment has substantial risks or side effects, but, as indicated above, there are also substantial risks in not treating this form of epilepsy. Clearly we do not understand the reason for the related retardation or its optimal treatment. Further research is needed.

## Lennox-Gastaut Syndrome

The Lennox-Gastaut syndrome, named after the two epileptologists who described its various components, is characterized by two or more types of seizures, one of which is the atonic (falling down) type; by a particular EEG pattern of diffuse spike or poly-spike and slow waves; and by mental retardation.

The syndrome usually begins between the ages of two and six and in more than one-third of the cases evolves in children who previously had infantile spasms. As with infantile spasms, there is no known single cause, but the syndrome commonly arises in children with developmental problems of the brain or acquired brain damage. A small percentage of these children appear to be normal before the seizures begin and have a later age of onset (cryptogenic). In this latter group, it is important to search for a degenerative process that may be causing the seizures. If none is present, this cryptogenic group may have a somewhat better prognosis than children whose seizures are symptomatic of a known disease process.

Children with the Lennox-Gastaut syndrome commonly experience multiple seizure types. In the most disabling seizures the child suddenly falls to the ground, either forward or less often backward, frequently injuring himself. Many of these children are forced to wear football helmets with face masks to protect their teeth and faces from trauma. In addition, tonic seizures and atypical absence seizures are common, with occasional tonic-clonic seizures as well.

Children with these multiple, difficult-to-control seizures often are given several simultaneous medications with consequent drug toxicity. The handicapping nature of the seizures, plus the drug toxicity and the continuous electrical abnormalities on the EEG, often reinforce the intrinsic brain dysfunction and produce a severely handicapped child.

Valproic acid has been the most effective anticonvulsant for children with this syndrome, and it should be used alone and in high doses as the initial drug. It may, if necessary, be supplemented by one of the other anticonvulsants for generalized tonic-clonic seizures or with a benzodiazepine.

We have found the ketogenic diet (see Chapter 12) also quite effective and recommend its use early in the course of the syndrome. We have had less success with the MCT diet. The effectiveness of oral steroids and ACTH also has been noted. The role of a form of surgery, corpus callosum sectioning (see Chapter 13), in young children with this syndrome is under investigation.

Clearly, as with infantile spasms, the Lennox-Gastaut syndrome is a most frustrating and devastating condition. This group of children make up a large proportion of the intractable seizure population. Research is badly needed to understand their condition and to develop better forms of therapy. The frustration involved in their management and the complexity of treatment lead us to suggest that these children be evaluated and managed under the consultation of sophisticated epilepsy centers with access to newer drugs.

### Neonatal Seizures

Seizures in the newborn are virtually always a consequence of metabolic causes, damage to the brain, or lack of oxygen, thus virtually always "symptomatic." Since they may or may not be associated with later epilepsy, they do not require long-term treatment unless other seizures recur.

## Special Conditions that Cause Epilepsy

Most children who have epilepsy do not have mental retardation, cerebral palsy, or other problems. Most children who do have mental retardation or cerebral palsy do not have epilepsy. However, sometimes brain damage due to lack of oxygen, head trauma, or problems of brain development may lead to both epilepsy and mental retardation or cerebral palsy.

Let us talk briefly about some of these special conditions.

## Developmental Abnormalities of the Brain

For reasons that are presently unclear, abnormalities in brain development can result in seizures. The development of the brain is a series of events in which cells move and interconnections are established so complex that it amazes and awes physicians. Many different abnormalities can occur during this development; the cells may be too large, misconnected, or malformed, or they may not move to the proper place in the brain.

Most commonly abnormalities in brain development involve the entire brain; they tend to be accompanied by mental retardation and cerebral palsy. On occasion, these abnormalities may be focal and produce focal seizures. Such abnormalities may be surgically treated if that area of the brain can be safely removed. Less commonly, these developmental abnormalities may involve only one half of the brain, resulting in paralysis of one side of the body and unilateral seizures. If such a child has uncontrollable seizures, removal of that abnormal half of the brain (hemispherectomy) may be a life-saving and seizure-curing procedure (Chapter 13).

### Tuberous Sclerosis

Tuberous sclerosis is an inherited condition in which children may have white birthmarks on their skin and other skin lesions, mental retardation, and epilepsy. There is an abnormality of cell development affecting many organs of the body. In the brain, cells may be abnormal and may form small tumors. The cellular abnormalities and tumors, in turn, may cause epilepsy, either focal or generalized. The most common form of epilepsy is infantile spasms, discussed above. A diagnosis of tuberous sclerosis is indicated if multiple white spots (see Fig. 8.1) appear on the skin. Older children may develop acne-like changes on their faces. The CT or MRI scan may show the tumors or areas of calcification.

The outcome of children with tuberous sclerosis varies, as does the epilepsy. Some individuals may be of normal intelligence with no significant problems. Others may have substantial mental retardation and seizures difficult to control.

If your child has this condition, it is important to talk with your physician about the possibility that your other children may also be affected.

## Neurofibromatosis

Neurofibromatosis is also an inherited condition involving many organ systems and with skin abnormalities consisting of multiple brown birth marks ("cafe-au-lait spots") (see Fig. 8.2). As with tuberous sclerosis, abnormalities of cell development within the brain may cause mild mental retardation and seizures. Tumors may occur on nerves, creating pressure on the surrounding nervous system tissue, leading to paralysis and other disabling conditions. Your doctor can discuss with you the many forms of this condition, their varying outcomes, as well as the genetic implications.

## Sturge-Weber Syndrome

Sturge-Weber syndrome is not inherited. It is an abnormality of blood vessel formation occurring early in the development of the fetal face and brain. Children with this disease are born with a red birthmark ("port wine stain") on the forehead and, at times, extending over the eye and lower face (Fig. 8.3A, B). Birthmarks that do not appear on the forehead are not associated with Sturge-Weber syndrome.

In this disease, blood vessel malformation causes atrophy (shrinking) of the underlying brain, leading to seizures and paralysis of the opposite side of the body. The seizures that accompany this shrinkage are usually one-sided and may be difficult to control with medication. Children with Sturge-Weber syndrome may be of normal intelligence but are often progressively handicapped by mental retardation, by the seizures, and by paralysis. Surgery to remove the affected portion of the brain is sometimes indicated and should be done early in treatment.

Laser surgery for the facial birthmark (hemangioma) shows promise of alleviating this disfiguring problem.

## Chronic Infections

Acute bacterial and viral infections of the brain (meningitis and encephalitis), as we know, may cause acute seizures and may occasionally damage the brain and result in epilepsy. Other infections that occur before birth or, rarely, after birth may also damage the brain and lead to epilepsy. The most common infection of the brain world-wide is cysticercosis; in some countries this may be the most common cause of epilepsy, but in the United States it is a rare cause of seizures. A doctor will suspect this diagnosis when single or multiple areas of typical

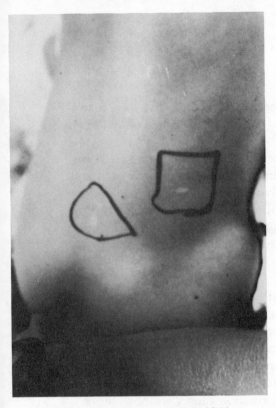

**Figure 8.1.** Tuberous sclerosis. Multiple white spots, subtle and ash-leaf in shape.

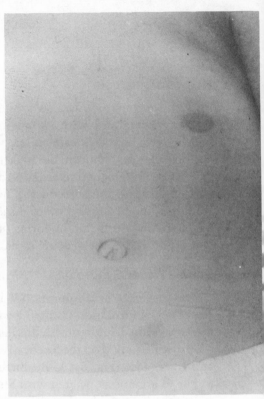

**Figure 8.2.** Neurofibromatosis. *Cafe-au-lait,* brownish and multiple.

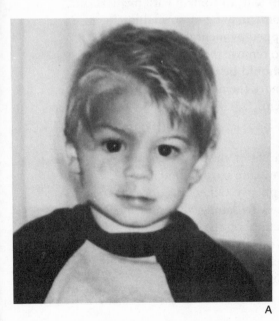

A

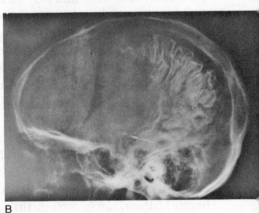

B

**Figure 8.3.** Sturge-Weber disease. Note the birthmark over the child's right forehead, eye, and lip (A); x-ray of the skull of a child with Sturge-Weber disease (B), with calcifications of the brain in a classic railroad-track pattern.

calcification, the result of cysts within the brain, are spotted on the CT. Surgical removal of these cysts may cure the child's epilepsy.

Another brain infection is toxoplasmosis, an infection spread by cats. If a pregnant woman acquires this infection it may be transmitted to her baby and cause scarring in the brain. Infection, often undetectable in the newborn, is first manifested, possibly, as mental retardation or as seizures. A CT scan can detect scars within the brain and aid diagnosis. Also, small scars on the retina in back of the eye may be noted by your physician and suggest a diagnosis. In addition, blood tests can confirm what the observations suggest. Suspected toxoplasmosis is often treated in an attempt to prevent further damage. The treatment of seizures in affected children is similar to those used in the treatment of other forms of epilepsy.

## Herpes Virus

Herpes simplex virus is a common human infection. It takes two forms. One is the cold sore which occurs around the mouth. This form (herpes type I) rarely affects the brain. Herpes type II affects the genital region. A baby born to a woman whose cervix is actively infected may, in turn, acquire the virus, which may devastate its brain, producing severe retardation, cerebral palsy, and epilepsy. In addition, a brain infection caused by the herpes simplex type II virus may be acquired at any age and produce complex partial seizures and an overwhelming encephalitis. Early detection may enable treatment to be more effective. Babies who survive have variable degrees of brain damage and epilepsy.

## HIV Infections (AIDS)

AIDS is a growing problem for infants born to human immuno-deficiency (HIV)-infected mothers and children who acquire AIDS from transfusion, drug abuse, and sexual activity. The HIV virus affects the brain and may produce seizures. The multiple infections that are byproducts of the immunosuppression due to AIDS may also affect the brain and cause seizures. Secondary infections require specific treatment, but the seizures are treated with standard anticonvulsant medication.

## Rasmussen's Syndrome

A rare form of progressive unilateral seizures, usually associated with a progressive weakness of one side of the body, has been termed

Rasmussen's encephalitis, in honor of the Canadian neurosurgeon who first described it. While the pathologic changes in the brain suggest a viral cause, no virus has ever been found, however, and the cause of this condition remains unknown.

The progressive nature of a disorder that seems to be "eating away the brain" and that causes seizures growing in severity and slowly increasing neurologic decline may suggest this diagnosis to your physician. Brain scans may indicate progressive shrinkage in the affected areas. Anticonvulsant medication is rarely effective in controlling the seizures, nor does surgical removal of the most affected parts of the brain halt the progression of the disease throughout the single hemisphere. However, this peculiar condition does seem to be limited to one half of the brain, and therefore, if surgical removal of that half of the brain by hemispherectomy is undertaken early, it usually abolishes seizures and permits normal intellectual development. There will be paralysis on the affected side, but without surgery the consequences are worse.

### Degenerative Diseases

A number of progressive, degenerative diseases of the brain affect children. Epilepsy is commonly seen in most of them. One group is called storage diseases because the proteins and fats that are normally broken down to waste products (metabolized) and eliminated from the body cannot be broken down in these rare inherited metabolic conditions. These products accumulate within nerve cells and affect their function, leading to epilepsy and mental retardation. These progressive conditions are usually fatal, but the duration of the illness may be quite variable. The names attached to these storage diseases reflect the individuals who described the conditions and the material stored. Different conditions begin at different ages. Among these conditions are Tay-Sachs disease (GM2 gangliosidosis), Batten's disease (ceroid lipofuscinosis), and the various leukodystrophies. In the leukodystrophies, epilepsy is likely to appear later in the course of the progressive disease.

Although many of the epilepsy syndromes and some of these infections sound very frightening and can be devastating to both the child and the family, fortunately these conditions are uncommon. Most children with epilepsy do not have these conditions and their seizures are controlled. Most children with epilepsy do very well.

# Part Three

# Treating Seizures and Epilepsy

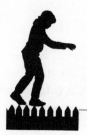

# 9. Medical Treatment of Seizures

## Philosophy of Treatment

Although once it was believed that all seizures should be treated, just because they were there, now it is generally believed that no judgment can cover every individual. Decisions about treatment should be made by the patient (or parent) *and* the physician acting in partnership. The decision should be based on risk-benefit analysis.

The risks and consequences of each medication vary with the medicine, with the dose, with the individual's reaction to the medicine, with the age of the child, and with the length of time the child takes the medicine. The risk of further seizures varies markedly with the type of seizure, the frequency of seizures, and even the time of day in which they occur. A child who has only occasional tonic-clonic seizures at night will face very different risks from a child whose seizures occur during the day. A child with occasional complex partial seizures has different risks from the child with tonic-clonic seizures or the child with frequent absence seizures.

Most people's seizures can be controlled with a single medicine used in a proper dose to achieve a proper blood level for that individual. *There is no correct dose of a given medication.* The "proper" dose of medication is the dose that completely controls the seizures without causing significant side effects. *There is not a "correct" medication as such. Some medicines work better for some types of seizures than for others. The correct medicine is the one that works.*

*The treatment of epilepsy is empirical.* This means that the treatment of each person's seizures is a trial or search to find the appropriate dose

**119**

of the best medicine for that individual. This "experimentation" is often frustrating to parents since they are used to physicians' knowing, for example, the right antibiotic and dose to use for a child's ear infection.

For drugs like antibiotics, we know how they act, the proper dose, and the side effects. We know how much is necessary to kill the bacteria causing the infection. We can test the drug's effectiveness in the laboratory. We know, for example, how "heart drugs" work and their side effects, we can use the electrocardiogram (EKG) to see if they are working or if they are producing toxicity. But, since we do not fully understand how anticonvulsant drugs work, and since we do not understand the factors that permit a seizure to occur at a specific time, each child must be his own laboratory as a doctor attempts to find the proper dose of the best anticonvulsant. Side effects will vary with each child's metabolism and his individual reaction to the drug.

## How Anticonvulsant Drugs Work in Epilepsy

In an ideal world, we would understand the chemistry and the physiologic mechanisms causing epilepsy—how cells interact, fire, and misfire. Then we would design drugs that interact with the brain and prevent the misfiring, the seizures, without affecting the brain's normal function. As we have previously indicated, we do not know how or why a seizure occurs. While we have many drugs that are effective in treating and preventing seizures, we do not know how they work.

Because epilepsy is a result of complex interactions in the brain, and since these interactions cannot be accurately simulated in a test tube or by a computer, animal experimentation has been necessary for us to understand epilepsy and learn how to control it. Most anticonvulsants were discovered by experimenting with substances to see if they would work in animals that had seizures caused by certain drugs. Such animal seizures, although not the same as epilepsy, have many similarities. Such research has been highly useful, and it must continue.

Although we do not know how the drugs work, we do know a lot about how they are absorbed and metabolized in the body and about their side effects. This knowledge enables us to use them properly, to calculate a dose, and to predict effects and side effects. This knowledge is called the pharmacology of the drugs; your physician will use this knowledge in treating your child and controlling her seizures.

## Terms You Need to Know

*Drug levels.* The term "drug level" refers to the amount of a medication in the blood—to be more precise, the serum levels, since the drug is in the liquid portion of your blood (serum) rather than in the red blood cells. To be still more precise, we should refer to the amount of "free" drug in the serum, since virtually all of a drug is tightly bound to the proteins in the serum and cannot get into the brain to exert its effect; only the tiny "free" (unbound) portion can enter the brain to affect the seizures. When we measure "drug levels" or "blood levels," we usually measure the total amount of a drug in the serum. In most cases this is sufficient, but we can, when necessary, measure the free portion as well, although it is a somewhat more expensive test. In general, when we talk about drug levels in this chapter, we are referring to serum levels.

*Toxicity.* The term "toxicity" covers a multitude of things. Toxicity, in general, is used here to refer to the adverse (bad) effects of a medication. There are two major forms of such toxicity: allergic and dose-related. The allergic form may be mild (such as a rash) or severe, affecting the blood cells, bone marrow, or liver, reactions that can be serious and, rarely, even fatal. The dose-related form depends on the amount of medication in the brain. Toxicity may be observed as sleepiness (sedation), unsteadiness (ataxia), tremor, or even as problems in learning. Dose-related toxicities are important to recognize, and when recognized are seldom serious, because they are reversible by a decreasing or a discontinuing of the drug.

*Half-life.* This is the amount of time it takes for one half of the drug in the body to be metabolized (broken down) or to be excreted. Therefore, if a dose of a medicine reaches a level of 10 in your body, that drug's half-life is the amount of time it takes until the blood level decreases to 5. This is important to you because the half-life for some drugs is only a few hours but for others it may be days. A drug's half-life will determine how often your child must take his medicine—one, two, or even four times per day. The half-life varies with each drug and with the age of the child.

As an example: We start your child on drug A, which has a half-life of twelve hours. We tell you to give the two daily doses twelve hours apart. If your child's drug level was 20 one hour after a dose, it would fall to 10 just before the next dose. If 10 were too low to control your child's seizures, she might have a seizure before the evening dose. If we gave the same dose, but told you to give the medicine every eight hours, then eight hours after a dose the level might be 14, and that might be sufficient to prevent a seizure (Fig. 9.1).

*Steady state.* In general, it takes five half-lives to achieve a steady state of a relatively consistent blood level of a drug between doses (Fig. 9.2). After one dose of a medicine, let's say that the blood level is 8. One half-life later the level has decreased. If a second dose is then given, the blood level rises. You can see that the blood level is slowly creeping up. If you continue this process, then after five half-lives there is insignificant change in the blood level between doses.

You must allow each new medication sufficient time to achieve a steady state before you know if is going to work. For example, since phenobarbital has a half-life of three days, it will take at least two weeks to achieve its new steady state. If your child has a seizure five days after starting phenobarbital, or after increasing the dose, it may not mean that the drug will not work. It means rather that there hasn't been enough time to test that dose of the drug. You have to be patient.

*After a new steady-state is achieved you will have to allow sufficient time to know if the new level will control seizures. As a general rule, each new drug and each new dose of a drug should be given a trial of at least seven to fourteen days before a change is considered.*

An exception to this rule may occur when the child is having seizures daily or several times each day. Then you may not want to wait two weeks or even one before changing the dose. In this situation, your physician can "load" the child with the drug. This means if she wishes to achieve a high, consistent blood level more rapidly, she can give more of the drug, usually two to three times as much as usual. This will produce an initially high level and may cause substantial temporary side effects.

The side effects of medication are related to both the level of medication in the blood and to the brain's individual reaction. The brain will often become accustomed to a drug. Many people feel sleepy when first started on a medication, but after several weeks, they may become "used" to it and be normally alert.

A second application of the concept of half-life is this: Let's say your child is taking phenytoin (Dilantin) and accidentally took too many pills. You become concerned when you find him very unsteady, acting as if he were drunk. When you discover the overdose and call your physician, she is likely to say, "Don't worry, it will wear off. We have to let it

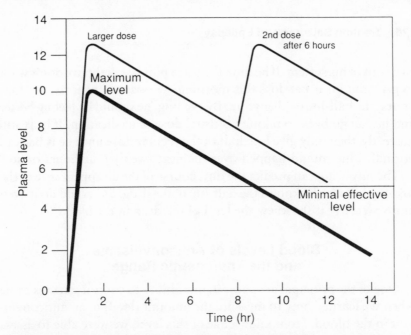

**Figure 9.1.** Half-life of a drug. Drugs are absorbed at different rates. As shown in the figure, the drug taken by mouth takes approximately an hour to reach its maximum blood (plasma) level of 10, then is slowly metabolized and excreted. The amount in the blood falls to half of its maximum level (5) eight hours later; thus, the half-life of this drug is eight hours. If a second dose were to be given six hours after the first, the body would be absorbing new medicine and the blood level would never fall below the minimum effective level for preventing seizures.

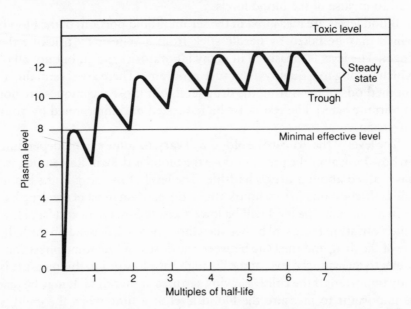

**Figure 9.2.** Steady-state. Steady-state is reached at point when there is relatively little fluctuation in the level of a drug in the body; in general, it takes five half-lives to reach the steady-state.

clear out of his system. If he took the extra pills last night, we don't want to give him his usual dose this morning. We want to wait twenty-four hours, the half-life of phenytoin. By evening, he should be feeling better and he can go back to taking his usual dose of medication. If he is still unsteady, then only give him half of the regular dose until he is back to normal. This should happen over the next twenty-four hours or so."

The physician can predict the time course of the disappearance of the toxicity because he knows the half-life of the drug. She could do it even more precisely if she knew the level of the drug in the blood.

## Blood Levels of Anticonvulsants and the Therapeutic Range

One of the principal advances in our ability to control seizures came when we learned how to measure the amount (level) of an anticonvulsant in the blood. From knowledge of this level, we were able to assess the amount of the drug actually reaching the brain. And yet this advance is less than two decades old.

Even now many physicians do not fully understand the use of blood levels and the concept of the "therapeutic range" of a given drug. Parents (and physicians) often believe that these levels ensure control of the seizures or guarantee the absence of side effects, misbeliefs that often lead to misuse of the blood levels.

Blood levels are measured in the serum (liquid portion) of the blood, which may be taken by needle stick from a vein or by pricking the finger. The level is measured in many laboratories, most, but not all of which belong to a quality assurance program. (There are several different methods of measuring the drug level, but those techniques are not important here.) The test must be requested and interpreted by your physician.

The level of the drug in the blood will vary, to some extent, depending on how long after the previous dose the blood is drawn. Remember, we have talked about a drug's half-life. The level of the drug in the blood will be highest one to two hours after a dose, when most of the drug has been absorbed. The level will be lowest just before the next dose. How much variation there will be between those two will depend on the half-life of the drug and the time between the doses. While some physicians prefer to measure the level at the "trough," the low point, this measure is only important if the child is having seizures at that time. It may be just as important to measure the blood level at a time when the child is

Table 9.1    Pharmacological Facts for Selected Antiepileptic Drugs

| Drug | Daily dosage range (mg/kg/day) | Serum therapeutic range (μg/Ml) | Half-life (hr) | Time to reach stable levels (wk) |
|------|------|------|------|------|
| Carbamazepine (Tegretol) | 10–25 | 4–12 | 10–30 | 1 |
| Ethosuximide (Zarontin) | 10–70 | 45–100 | 24–42 | 1–2 |
| Phenobarbital | 1–5 | 10–20 | 30–150 | 2–3 |
| Phenytoin (Dilantin) | 4–12 | 10–20 | 3–60 | 2 |
| Primidone (Mysoline) | 10–20 | 8–20 | 6–8 | 2–3 |
| Valproic acid (Depakote) | 10–70 | 50–100 | 4–15 | $1/2$ |

*Note:* Names of drugs that appear in parentheses are brand names; others are generic names.

having seizures to see if the level is low, or to measure it when the child is sleepy, dizzy, or having other unexplained symptoms in order to ensure that the level is not too high.

*What is the correct blood level for your child? The correct blood level is the amount of the drug that controls the seizures. It is not a specific amount. The optimal level is the lowest level that works without causing toxicity. It will vary from one child to another.*

This brings us to the concept of "the therapeutic range," a concept often misunderstood. Therapeutic ranges for the commonly used anticonvulsants are shown in Table 9.1. It may be useful to understand how the therapeutic ranges for these drugs have been established. A small number of adults (or children) were carefully studied using a single drug. The lower end of the therapeutic range was then determined by the level at which seizures begin to be controlled in a majority of these individuals. The upper end of the range was the point at which some individuals began to show signs of toxicity. Thus, the *"therapeutic range"* is the drug level at which most individuals are likely to be controlled without toxicity. Your child is not an average but an individual. Thus he or she may require a more-than-average level, or a less-than-average level to control the seizures. He may be able to tolerate more or less than average levels before showing signs of toxicity. Therefore, finding the correct dose of a given drug for your child requires a trial to determine what is "enough" and what is "too much" for *your* child.

The therapeutic range is commonly believed to be the "gold standard" that will guarantee seizure control and avoid toxicity and side effects. It does neither. Yet many physicians misinterpret the therapeutic range as the range where they should keep the blood level, decreasing the dose of the medicine if the blood level is above the range and increasing it if the level is below the range.

*To repeat, the correct blood level for your child is enough—enough to control the seizures and not enough to cause toxicity. The therapeutic range is a guide, nothing more.*

## Common Questions about Blood Levels

Physicians and parents have become enamored of tests and often give them greater importance than is proper. Despite scientific advances, the proper use of anticonvulsants remains an art, not always a science. We are often asked questions by both physicians and parents.

### *"My doctor says that my child's blood level is slightly low and wants to increase his dose. What should I do?"*

If you ask us this, we would ask if your child is still having seizures. If he is, then the dose should be increased. If he is not, then we would leave the dose alone; the current level may be sufficient to control his seizures. The question of increasing a dose often comes up in a child whose seizures are controlled. As the child grows and increases in size, the blood level will, of course, decrease if your doctor doesn't increase the dose. But we suggest keeping the dose the same as the child grows and gains weight, unless he is having seizures. If the dose is kept the same, then the blood level gradually falls over the months or years. If the child does not have another seizure, it will be easier and safer to take him off his medicine when he has been free of seizures for two years. If he has a seizure, then you know that he needs to stay on the medication longer.

*"My daughter's blood level is at the upper end of 'normal,' and she is still having seizures. My doctor wants to try another drug. Is that the proper thing to do?"*

We would suggest first that he try increasing the dose even further, but slowly, since your daughter is close to the point where many people show toxicity. Sometimes seizures will be controlled with a little more drug without any toxic problems. The upper level of the therapeutic range is like a sign post, "WARNING"; it suggests that you and your physician should be watchful for signs of toxicity.

*"Rachel's blood level is 'high,' and my doctor wants to lower the dose. I think that she is doing just fine, and she hasn't had any seizures since that last increase in dosage. What should we do?"*

We would recommend that you leave the dose alone. If Rachel isn't having any seizures and has no signs of toxicity, then perhaps this is the level she requires. However, since the level is above the usual range, we would suggest that you keep a close eye on her and on her school performance to be sure that the drug is not interfering and that you stay alert for other signs of toxicity.

*"Billy's blood level is right in the middle of the 'range.' Is that good?"*

The answer to this question is, "It depends." If Billy is not having any seizures and shows no signs of toxicity, then that level is fine and should not be changed. If he is still having seizures, then the level is too low for him, and he needs more medication. If he is too sleepy, too irritable, or having problems in school, then it is important to find out why. There are many causes for problems such as these. Obviously, you should be sure that he is not having seizures. If the level is not high, then the drug is a less likely cause. However, if you can't find another cause, then lowering or discontinuing the drug may be worth trying. If the problem disappears, then it may have been due to the drug.

*To summarize, the therapeutic range is a guide and nothing more. It will suggest to you and your physician when it may be appropriate to increase the drug and when to look more closely for signs of toxicity. The range does not tell you when the child is taking too much or too little. Control of seizures and signs of toxicity are the only things that tell that.*

*"Trudy has been on phenobarbital but is continuing to have seizures. Your doctor starts her on valproic acid, but several days later she is very sleepy and unsteady. Why?"*

You and your physician might assume that she is toxic from the new medicine, but you would probably be wrong. A blood level might show you that the valproate level was actually low, but that the phenobarbital level had now increased to the toxic range, and that phenobarbital was the true offender. This effect is due to what we call "drug interactions"—one drug interfering with the breakdown or metabolism of another. Drug interactions are common; some decrease the level of the other drug; some, like the valproate, increase the level of another. The only way you can be sure is by measuring each drug's blood level. Other medications, such as antibiotics or ulcer medications, to name a few, may also interact with anticonvulsants and alter levels.

While we talk about blood levels of a drug as if they were very important for control of seizures, *it is not the drug in the blood that is important, but rather the amount of the drug in the brain,* which is where these drugs work. However, we cannot easily measure the level of the drug in the brain, so we use the blood (serum) level as an approximation.

Most drugs are tightly bound to the proteins in the blood; this is the way they are carried around the body. They cannot get into the brain when they are bound up. Only the small amount of any drug which is not bound to protein (the "free" drug) enters the brain and is actually active. Usually when we measure the blood level, the test measures all of the drug in the blood, both bound and unbound. However, in special circumstances, such as a low serum protein level, when certain other drugs are present, or when there is severe kidney disease, more of the drug may be unbound and thus active. It is possible, and sometimes useful, to measure the "unbound" fraction, but most of the time we do not measure the unbound fraction of the drug because it requires a somewhat more difficult and, therefore, more expensive procedure.

*"How frequently does my child need to have his blood level measured?"*

We measure blood levels about two to three weeks after we start a new drug or change a dose to assure that we have the drug level in the range we had expected and that the child is not near the toxic range. If there are signs of toxicity, especially if the child is on more than one drug, we use the blood level to determine if the toxicity is caused by the drug and which drug should be decreased. We measure the level if the child is continuing to have seizures to see where in the "range" we are and to determine how much we should increase the dose. If the child is doing well, with seizures under control and without toxicity, we measure the level once or twice a year to assure that nothing has changed and that the child is taking the drug regularly. The medical community calls this consistency in taking medication "compliance." Lack of compliance, "non-compliance," is a major factor in recurrent seizures. Measuring the level occasionally when the child is doing well enables us to know what level is effective for controlling seizures in that child.

### *"My child's blood level of his medication is low. Why?"*

There are several possible reasons, perhaps the most common that the child is not on a high enough dose, a second that she is not receiving enough medication or is not taking the medicine. Non-compliance is a common reason for a low blood level, particularly among adolescents. Occasionally also an individual absorbs medicine poorly and must take more to achieve the same blood level. Rarely, an individual metabolizes the drug more rapidly than average and, therefore, has a low level. Whatever the reason, increasing the dose should help to determine the answer. If the person is taking the drug erratically or not at all, then prescribing more will usually have little or no effect. If the dose prescribed is too low, a higher dose should correct the problem, as it will do if the patient absorbs poorly or metabolizes rapidly.

*Your child does not necessarily need a blood level test every time he visits the doctor!*

### *"Sally had several grand mal seizures and was placed on a medicine. She has had no more seizures since age three, but she has grown and gained weight. Her physician finds that Sally's blood level has slipped below the 'therapeutic' range. What should he do?"*

This question of maintaining the level over time also needs to be addressed. In Sally's case there are two alternatives. The physician could increase the dose, and thus the blood level, to keep it in the therapeutic range giving her greater protection against another seizure. Or he could leave the dose alone, let it gradually continue to decrease as she grows, and when she has been free of seizures for two years, then he can discontinue the medicine. There is not, however, necessarily a correct thing to do. Children who have been free of seizures for two years can discontinue medication with a high probability of remaining seizure free. That chance is higher if the blood levels are low at the time the medicine is stopped because a child who is sensitive to the level of medication is more likely to have a seizure when the level drops below the therapeutic range. Then the doctor increases the dose and waits another two years. If the child is unlikely to have another seizure, then it doesn't matter if the blood level is low. Allowing the level to drop slowly is a form of testing. If Sally passes the test, her chance of having a seizure when we stop the medicine is low. If she fails the test and has another seizure, we believe that it is better for this to happen at a younger age. Therefore, our suggestion to this parent and this physician would be not to increase the medicine. We believe that the risks and consequences of another seizure at this age are outweighed by the possible side effects of a higher dose on Sally's learning capacity. Other physicians (and other parents) may believe differently.

## Choosing the Best Medication

All drugs do not work equally well for every seizure-type. Therefore it is necessary to classify the child's seizure. For each seizure-type there are several drugs that are usually equally effective. The choice between the drugs is then made on the basis of the drug's side effects and cost, the child's age, and any previous drug allergies. Some medications are more effective for partial and tonic-clonic seizures, others for absence seizures. We will discuss them in those groupings and the order in which they were discovered.

Commonly-used anticonvulsant medications and the types of seizure for which they are most often used are shown in Table 9.2. A large number of anticonvulsant medications are available. The following are those most commonly used.

## Drugs for Partial Seizures and Tonic-Clonic Seizures

### Phenobarbital

Phenobarbital is one of the oldest, cheapest, and safest of the anticonvulsants. Since phenobarbital is slowly metabolized by the body (has a long half-life), it usually can be taken only once per day. As with any drug, it can lead to occasional allergic reactions.

**Table 9.2    Use of Specific Anticonvulsant Drugs in Different Seizure Types**

|  | Partial (focal) | Absence | Tonic-clonic |
|---|---|---|---|
| Carbamazepine (Tegretol) | + |  | + |
| Clonazepam (Klonopin) |  | + | + |
| Clorazepate (Tranxene) | + | + | + |
| Ethosuximide (Zarontin) |  | + |  |
| Phenobarbital | + |  | + |
| Phenytoin (Dilantin) | + |  | + |
| Primidone (Mysoline) | + |  | + |
| Valproic acid (Depakote) | + | + | + |

*Note:* Names of drugs that appear in parentheses are brand names; others are generic names.

Phenobarbital, like its two close barbiturate cousins, mephobarbital (Mebaral) and primidone (Mysoline), is effective in partial and generalized tonic-clonic seizures but ineffective in absence seizures (and, indeed, may even cause them to increase).

### Reactions to phenobarbital and other barbiturate drugs

A skin rash may be the first sign of an allergic reaction to phenobarbital (or to any other drug). A child who develops a skin rash during the first two to three weeks of treatment with any anticonvulsant should immediately be seen by his physician. While most such rashes are NOT caused by the drug, continuing the drug in a child who is allergic to it may lead to severe and even fatal consequences.

Side effects that are dose-related are seen in certain children. The most important side effects of phenobarbital in children are its impacts on learning and behavior. While these side effects can occur in any child if the blood level is sufficiently high, certain individuals may react adversely even at "normal" blood levels.

Phenobarbital can also cause sedation (sleepiness). Many children become tolerant of this tired feeling. In others, the tired feeling continues and they do not tolerate the drug. Giving phenobarbital at bedtime may help to minimize this problem. Disturbances of sleep also can occur from use of the drug.

*Hyperactivity,* a behavioral side effect, may occur in 20 to 40 percent of young children taking phenobarbital. Hyperactivity is more common in children who were quite active to begin with. In one study, more than half of the children had to be taken off this drug because of the side effects of irritability and behavior problems.

Effects of phenobarbital on a child's *learning ability* may be its most disturbing side effect. These symptoms may be subtle and difficult to recognize and may account for some of the learning problems previously attributed to epilepsy itself. Most, perhaps all of these side effects are thought to disappear when phenobarbital is discontinued. Recent studies have also found an increased incidence of depression in adolescents who take phenobarbital, perhaps more frequent when there is a family history of depression. In some children, a depression thought to be caused by an emotional reaction to having epilepsy disappears when another medication is substituted for phenobarbital.

*We prefer, for all these reasons, not to use phenobarbital when alternative drugs are available, especially because of our concern about its effects on learning and behavior in the vulnerable young child. When we do use it, we carefully monitor the child's behavior and school performance.*

### Mephobarbital (Mebaral)

Mephobarbital is said to cause less hyperactivity than phenobarbital, but its effectiveness as an anticonvulsant and its effects on learning have been less well studied.

### Primidone (Mysoline)

Primidone is an effective anticonvulsant that is metabolized by the body into phenobarbital. Although the drug has not been well studied in children, hyperactivity and behavior problems have been observed. As with phenobarbital, a child on primidone should be carefully monitored for learning and behavior problems. Primidone must be started at a low dose and increased slowly over several weeks to avoid major problems with sedation and personality change.

### Phenytoin (Dilantin)

Phenytoin, a generic (non-brand) name for Dilantin, an excellent anticonvulsant that has been used for many years, is particularly effective for partial and generalized tonic-clonic seizures. Phenytoin also produces side effects, allergic and dose-related.

### Allergic reactions

As with phenobarbital, a skin rash may be the first sign of an allergic reaction to phenytoin. *A child who develops a skin rash during the first two to three weeks after starting phenytoin should be seen by his physician immediately.* Other, more severe "allergic" reactions to phenytoin may affect the liver or the bone marrow, although these reactions are rare.

### Dose-related reactions

The earliest sign of a high blood level of phenytoin is nystagmus (jerky movements of the eyes), a sign of no consequence since it does not interfere with vision or function and, therefore, does not require lowering the dose of the drug. Noticing it may be useful to your physician since it indicates that the drug is in a "good" therapeutic range. If, with the onset of an even higher blood level, the child begins to be unsteady on his feet and awkward with his hands, to act drunk, you should notify your physician. He will usually reduce the dose. Sleepiness or exaggeration of the "drunkenness" follow if the blood level goes even higher. Vomiting may also occur. All of these signs disappear over several days (several half-lives) if the dose is reduced.

Because phenytoin has an unusual metabolism, when its level in the blood is in the therapeutic range, small increases in dosage can cause large increases in the blood level and, thus, in toxicity. Therefore, when the blood level is in the therapeutic range but the dose must be increased to control seizures, increases should be introduced slowly and by small increments or the child may become toxic.

### Other side effects

Phenytoin also affects behavior and learning. The child's mood may change, and she may seem to have less energy. The child's motor abilities and her alacrity in performing tasks may also be affected. Hyperactivity is less common than with phenobarbital, however, and the effects on learning may be less severe than with phenobarbital.

Some of the dose-related side effects of phenytoin are cosmetic, that is, they affect the appearance of the child. Gum hyperplasia (overgrowth of the gums) occurs in almost one-half of the children who have therapeutic blood levels. The overgrowth is made much worse by poor dental hygiene; thus, when children are wearing braces gum overgrowth becomes an even more severe problem. *Children taking phenytoin should be taught good tooth-brushing techniques, and young children should have their teeth brushed by their parents. Good hygiene will diminish the gum swelling but not necessarily prevent it entirely.* Overgrown gums can be cut back by the dentist. Overgrowth of the gums may make secondary teeth come in with wide spaces and may later require extensive orthodontic care.

Children who have been on high doses of phenytoin for long periods of time often develop coarse facial features and more extensive body hair. The hair does not disappear when the drug is discontinued, although it may decrease. Such a side effect may become a cosmetic problem, especially for young women. *Although phenytoin is an excellent anticonvulsant, we prefer not to use it as our* initial *drug in young children because of its cosmetic side effects.* The cosmetic effects seem to be a lesser problem with adolescents and adults.

## Carbamazepine (Tegretol)

Carbamazepine is an excellent anticonvulsant medication for partial and generalized tonic-clonic seizures, and our initial choice for children with these seizures because of its apparent lower incidence of effects on learning and behavior and its lack of cosmetic side effects. Earlier concerns about carbamazepine's effect on the blood and bone marrow seem to have been greatly overstated, especially for children.

Carbamazepine, a seemingly very safe and effective anticonvulsant, "induces its own metabolism." If we start a child on the amount of medication that he'll eventually need to control seizures, he'll become toxic, so we start slowly. The half-life is longer when the medication is first introduced into the body; the body's metabolism hasn't been induced, or "turned on," and the drug accumulates. Therefore, when starting carbamazepine, the drug should be begun at a low dose and increased each week for the first several weeks to reach and maintain the appropriate blood level.

### Side effects of carbamazepine

The side effect of carbamazepine that worries most parents (and physicians) is a decrease in the white blood cells, responsible for fighting infection. The normal white blood cell count is in the range of 5000–8000 cells. Children (or adults) who are taking carbamazepine often have lower white cell counts, perhaps 3000–5000. In one in ten such children, this lowering of the white count is temporary; it persists in only two percent. Usually this persistent low white cell count is of no consequence since the child is able to fight infections just as well as anyone else.

If your child has a low white count while on carbamazepine, don't panic. Sometimes your child's white count may be low from a viral infection. Your physician may want to repeat the count in five to seven days. If it has come back toward normal, the carbamazepine can be continued. If it has dropped further, the drug may need to be stopped temporarily. Stopping the drug suddenly may cause seizures to recur.

Aplastic anemia, in which the bone marrow stops producing blood cells, is a *very* rare but serious complication. We are aware of only a few reported cases in children. There appears to be no way to predict if a child will develop this condition. Frequent blood counts are expensive and painful and, besides, we have not found them useful.

### Allergic side effects

As with other anticonvulsants, a drug rash occurring within the first two to three weeks after starting carbamazepine is a potentially serious sign. A child with a rash beginning at this time should always be seen promptly by your physician, who can then decide whether to discontinue the drug. Rare effects on the liver, bone marrow, and blood clotting cells (platelets) have also been reported.

### Dose-related side effects

The signs of dose-related toxicity from carbamazepine are important because they are briefly experienced by almost everyone who uses it. The first sign of mild toxicity is double vision, sometimes accompanied by blurred vision or dizziness, most likely to occur one to two hours after a dose, when the amount of the drug in the blood is at its highest. Such symptoms last one to two hours, until the blood level decreases, not a serious side effect. If persistent and bothersome, your physician may want either to lower the dose or to spread out the medicine in more frequent, smaller doses.

More significant toxicity is displayed in unsteadiness, ataxia, sleepiness, or foggy thinking. These symptoms should be brought to the attention of your physician, who will want to check the blood level of the drug and perhaps change your child's dose. All of these symptoms disappear when the dosage is decreased or the drug is discontinued.

Because of carbamazepine's short half-life, physicians often recommend that it be taken three or even four times each day. We, and most patients, find that taking a drug this often is cumbersome, and that patients often forget to take some doses. We prescribe the drug to be taken only twice a day. We tell the patient (or the parent) to observe carefully if seizures occur before the next dose. If they do, then we assume that the blood level dropped too low or that the time between doses is too long and change the schedule to three or, infrequently, four times a day.

The other reason why we may decide to give the drug more often than twice a day is a patient's experience of signs or symptoms of toxicity shortly after taking a dose. This indicates that we have given too much at one time, and again we will instruct the patient to take a smaller dose of the drug three times a day. Using this approach, we have found that the seizures of most children can be controlled if they take carbamazepine only twice a day.

In children taking carbamazepine who are given erythromycin (an antibiotic often used in place of penicillin) for infection, high levels of carbamazepine and toxicity often develop. If your physician prescribes erythromycin, he may need to lower the dose of carbamazepine temporarily.

### Valproic Acid (Depakene, Depakote)

Although useful in treating partial seizures and tonic-clonic seizures, valproic acid is particularly useful for treating absence seizures and, therefore, is discussed in that group.

## Drugs for Absence and Other Generalized Seizures

### Ethosuximide (Zarontin)

Ethosuximide is very effective in simple absence seizures, but has no effect on partial seizures or on generalized tonic-clonic seizures.

Allergic side effects to ethosuximide include rashes, blood problems, and liver disease, but such complications are *very* infrequent. Dose-related toxicity is also uncommon, and the drug dose may be increased even when the blood level is well beyond the usual "therapeutic range." Occasionally, hyperactivity and effects on learning have been noted at high blood levels, but the data is, so far, inadequate.

*In general, ethosuximide seems to be well-tolerated, safe, and effective, and is our drug of choice for simple absence seizures.*

## Valproic Acid (Depakene, Depakote)

Valproic acid, the newest of our major anticonvulsant medications, and with a uniquely broad range of actions, is effective in tonic-clonic seizures as well as in absence seizures, complex partial seizures, and myoclonic seizures (see Table 9.2).

There is no universal agreement about how this drug should be used. Some experts note that valproic acid has a very short half-life and, therefore, recommend using it three or four times a day. These same experts recommend keeping the blood level above 90—100 micrograms/ml. We, and other experts, find this drug very different from the other anticonvulsants and that its effectiveness has little to do with the blood level. We find that it works better after the child has taken it for several weeks, and that it continues to work for several weeks after the drug is stopped. If necessary for seizure control, we recommend increasing the dose up to a fixed amount based on the child's weight (30—60 mg/kg), virtually ignoring the blood level but watching for toxicity. Which of these two groups of experts is correct remains to be determined.

### Allergic side effects of valproic acid

The most severe allergic reaction to valproic acid is a severe, sometimes fatal liver failure. Such a reaction occurs in one out of 800 children younger than two years of age, in one out of 7,000 children ages two to ten, and in fewer than one in 100,000 children older than ten who are also taking multiple other drugs. The risk is lower when valproic acid is the only drug in use.

*While valproic acid is, in general, a safe anticonvulsant drug, it should be used with great caution in children younger than two years of age, and then preferably as the only drug.*

Valproic acid may also cause severe, persistent abdominal pain, accompanied by nausea and vomiting (pancreatitis). It may cause a decrease in the blood's clotting cells (platelets) and thus in the body's ability to form blood clots. Because frequent tests of blood counts, bloodclotting, and of liver function are expensive and painful, and, in addition, will not predict whether your child will incur one of these problems tomorrow or next week, we do not perform them on a frequent or routine basis.

In general, we counsel parents that if their child is taking valproic acid and is ill for several days or has changes in behavior or school performance, they should ask their doctor if this could be due to the anticonvulsant.

*We caution parents that if their child who is taking valproic acid has persistent vomiting, yellow skin (jaundice), darkened urine, easy bruising, or a tendency to bleed from cuts, they should contact their physician immediately. Also, before any surgery, your surgeon should be informed that your child is taking valproic acid, so that the ability of his blood to clot can be evaluated and the surgeon can be prepared to prevent or stop excessive bleeding.*

In some children, valproic acid may cause an increase in the blood level of ammonia, leading to sleepiness, headache, nausea, or vomiting. Children with these symptoms should have a blood ammonia level test, and if the ammonia level is found to be elevated, the valproic acid dose should be decreased or the medication stopped.

Valproic acid itself rarely affects learning or behavior negatively. It seldom causes sleepiness. If these symptoms occur when the drug is started, they usually are a consequence of an increase in the level of some other drug the child is taking, particularly phenobarbital. Valproic acid increases the blood level of phenobarbital by 30 percent; thus, the dose of phenobarbital must be decreased by one-third when valproate is begun.

Valproic acid (Depakene) may be irritating to the stomach and cause nausea, vomiting, and a decrease in appetite. These symptoms decrease if the drug is taken along with meals. Depakote, a slightly different form of the drug, is said to have fewer effects on the stomach.

Weight gain, loss of appetite, and temporary loss of hair also occur in some individuals who are taking valproic acid.

*Although the list of side effects of valproate seems long, we repeat that it is an excellent anticonvulsant drug, and, if used properly, it is also very safe.*

### The Benzodiazepines (Diazepam, Clonazepam, Clorazepate, and Lorazepam)

Benzodiazepines are a class of anticonvulsants with a number of drugs. Diazepam (Valium) and lorazepam (Ativan) are commonly used to treat status epilepticus; clonazepam (Klonopin) and clorazepate

(Tranxene), diazepam (Valium), and lorazepam (Ativan) are also frequently used for long-term therapy. All of these drugs may be useful in absence seizures also, but they are most effective in myoclonic seizures, sometimes in drop attacks (atonic seizures), and also in complex partial seizures. Since these drugs generally cause sleepiness, both irritability and hyperactivity in young children, as well as personality changes in all ages, they tend to be used as "add-on drugs," that is, when other medications have not succeeded in controlling the seizures. Also, the brain often becomes tolerant of these drugs, so doses must continually be raised to maintain a beneficial effect.

Allergic and cosmetic side effects of the benzodiazepines are uncommon, but the other side effects greatly limit their usefulness.

## Generic or Brand-Name Drugs?

The rate of absorption of many anticonvulsants will vary with different manufacturers, and there may be some variation in their metabolism as well. Thus the blood level may vary. In a sensitive individual, small changes in blood level may either allow seizures or cause toxicity. Therefore, we strongly urge that children take the brand-name drug rather than the cheaper generic form, at least until the generic drugs become more standardized and consistent. We strongly urge also that you always stick to the form made by the same manufacturer. The only way that this can be done is to use the brand name drug.

*The choice of an antiepileptic drug must be individualized, taking into account the seizure type and concerns about possible side effects in a particular child. The pharmacology of these medications is important because it tells us how long we should expect to wait to see the impact of our therapy and how frequently the drug should be administered.*

*All medications have potential side effects, and parents should be familiar with the ones most commonly associated with the drug their child is taking. Monitoring the impact of therapy is crucial—whether seizures have been completely controlled and whether there are any unwanted side effects. It is always the response of the child that is important, not what the blood level is. Understandably, one-drug monotherapy is preferable to multi-drug polytherapy, and a concerted attempt at seizure control with a single drug should be made before another drug is added. Most seizures can be controlled in children using this careful approach, leading to the question of how long therapy should be continued.*

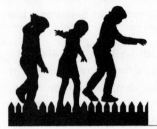

# 10. Status Epilepticus:
# A Medical Emergency

**"Suppose the seizure lasts more than 30 minutes. Suppose the child has one seizure after another without waking up between them. What do I do then?"**

STATUS EPILEPTICUS IS A MEDICAL EMERGENCY! "Status epilepticus" is defined as a seizure that lasts a long time. Some people define a long time as twenty minutes, thirty minutes, or an hour. We would recommend not being too concerned about a tonic-clonic "grand mal" seizure that lasts fewer than ten to fifteen or twenty minutes. There is no evidence that even thirty minutes of generalized tonic-clonic movement does damage to the brain. Even an hour of tonic-clonic seizures is unlikely to do damage to the brain, but we would *not* recommend purposely allowing a seizure to continue that long.

There are actually two types of status. One is the status epilepticus that most people think about, *convulsive status,* in which the patient is having tonic-clonic, shaking seizures for this long period of time. A separate type, *nonconvulsive status,* is an episode when a patient has absence spells, staring spells, or periods of confusion lasting a half-hour, an hour, or (rarely) days. This nonconvulsive status is not life-threatening or brain-damaging, but should be recognized.

## Convulsive Status Epilepticus and Its Treatment

Physicians are taught that a seizure lasting more than thirty minutes can do permanent damage to the brain. The medical literature says that as many as half of the patients with status epilepticus die or are left with permanent brain damage. But sometimes the things we think we know are not true!

Recent evidence suggests that it is not the seizures but the *cause* of the seizures that does the brain damage. Status epilepticus can be a consequence of infection of the brain, such as meningitis or encephalitis. It can be a consequence of head trauma, brain tumors, or other serious causes. When status epilepticus is "symptomatic"—due to something serious—usually it is the "something serious" that does damage to the brain *and* causes the status epilepticus. It is this *symptomatic* status that may result in death or permanent brain damage. Whether the seizures themselves cause further damage is much less clear.

Status epilepticus may occur as the first seizure a child experiences and in that case is often the *only* seizure he ever has. Whether the patient's first seizure is status or a brief, generalized, tonic-clonic seizure, most children (70 percent) never have another episode. Although there are many different causes of status epilepticus, *in most children the cause remains unknown*. When status epilepticus is of unknown cause or is part of a seizure disorder, it rarely causes permanent brain damage.

There are many causes of status epilepticus; whatever the cause, it is important to stop the prolonged seizures as promptly as possible. It is also crucial to evaluate each child and each episode of status to identify any underlying cause that may require specific treatment.

The treatment of status epilepticus is a task for skilled physicians, not for parents. But we're sure that you would like to know what the physicians are doing and why. First, they will take your child into a special place in the emergency room to make sure that he is breathing properly. They may give him oxygen by mask, suction saliva out of the throat, and observe him for a few minutes to see the seizures. While they are observing, they will draw some blood to check for infection and to check for the level of blood sugar and other chemicals in the body that could be out of balance and causing seizures. If your child has previously had seizures and is taking medicine, the physicians will want to check the blood for the level of the anticonvulsants. They may also check for any drugs or medications taken accidentally. They will start an intravenous line (IV) to introduce fluids and so that they can give anticonvulsant medications into the vein if necessary. Intravenous is the best way to give medications when a child is continuing to have seizures, because it is the most rapid way to get the medicine to the brain to stop the seizures. All of these things should take place in the first several minutes after arrival in the emergency room.

During this time the medical team also will take a brief history, searching for reasons for the status. They will be particularly concerned about any current illness, because meningitis or encephalitis, which could be a cause of the seizures, would require prompt treatment. The medical staff will want to know from you if the child has ever had seizures before, if there possibly has been an injury to the head, and things like that. Anything that you could think of that might have led the child to have a seizure *at this particular time* could be of help to the physicians.

If the seizures have been continuing more than fifteen, twenty, thirty minutes, the physicians will want to give medication to stop them. Various medications may be used, but drugs like diazepam (Valium) or lorazepam (Ativan), quick-acting effective anticonvulsants, are used initially. Unfortunately, although they work quickly, they often do not continue to work over a long period of time, and when they wear off— in ten to twenty minutes, or longer in the case of lorazepam—another seizure may occur. Therefore, the physician usually will give an additional drug, such as phenytoin (Dilantin), which works less quickly than the other but lasts longer.

If status epilepticus is the child's first seizure, then the doctors will probably want to do a lumbar puncture (spinal tap) to look for infection. They will study the blood for possible chemical changes and, perhaps, do an EEG then or the next day. They may even do a CT scan.

If the child has had other seizures or has epilepsy, then looking for a cause of the status may be slightly less important.

*The most common cause of status epilepticus in a person who has previously had seizures is that the level of medication in the blood is too low.* This may be because the child is not taking his medication, or that it has been forgotten, or that an interaction with some other medication has lowered the level. Substitution of a generic drug that is less well absorbed may also result in status epilepticus.

In almost all instances, the status epilepticus can be controlled within one-half hour to one hour from the time the child arrives in the emergency room and treatment is started. Only in an unusual situation, when there is an acute process occurring in the brain such as infection or damage from a head injury, do seizures continue, and are they difficult to control. Treatment of severe prolonged status epilepticus can be enormously challenging for the physician, requiring large doses of medication given in an intensive care unit and sometimes requiring general anesthesia to stop the seizures.

The outcome of status epilepticus, even in these severe episodes, depends more on the cause than on the duration of the seizures. Rest assured that most children who have status recover and are just as normal as they were before the seizures. It appears to be very, very rare for children who have status without a known cause to suffer any permanent damage, even from prolonged seizures.

## Nonconvulsive Status Epilepticus and Its Treatment

Just as there are many types of seizures, so there are diverse types of status epilepticus. Since these other types do not involve shaking, they are called nonconvulsive status epilepticus.

A child with petit mal seizures or absence seizures may just stop and stare and be unaware of his environment for brief episodes, lasting from a few seconds to a minute or two; these episodes are accompanied by spikes and waves on the EEG. On *rare* occasions, these seizures may continue for a long time, thirty minutes, an hour, occasionally even a day or two. This type of status is much harder to detect, since there is no shaking. The child may seem confused, or dull, or just quite different from his or her usual state. Sometimes there is confusion and the child seems lost, wandering around, unable to answer. On other occasions, a child acts as if his IQ had suddenly decreased twenty or thirty points. He or she may be able to answer you, but not with usual quickness or alertness. The child may appear dull, or just different. While there are many possible causes for this change, one cause could be that the child is in "nonconvulsive" status.

In addition to this suddenly altered state, the child may have brief eye blinks or staring or repetitive movements, but the only thing that may be different is that the child is not his usual self. When this state lasts for hours, when it is clear to you that something has suddenly changed, your physician should be consulted. The change could be due to medication or illness, it could be other drugs, it could be a different kind of illness, but *it could be nonconvulsive status.* How can you tell? The answer is, you can't. Even the physician can't necessarily tell from just looking at the child.

An EEG done during the episode is the only *certain* way to establish this nonconvulsive status diagnosis. The EEG usually shows constant spike-wave abnormalities that clearly interfere with cortical function, with thinking. If the EEG confirms the "spike-wave stupor" or nonconvulsive status, then the physician can give small amounts of medication (diazepam) in the vein; this will usually stop the brain wave abnormality abruptly and allow the child to return to normal.

☐ Joanne was a bright, sparkly second grader when we first met her. She was referred because of a "weird" episode the previous week. One day in school, she quite suddenly did not seem herself. She was quiet, wandered about the class, and responded inappropriately to the teacher. Her mother took her home, and after another hour or two, when she still wasn't herself, she had been taken to another hospital. No cause for the sudden change was found, but the next morning an EEG showed slowing, as if she might have previously had a seizure.

When we saw her the following week, she was fine and back to her usual self. Since she had never had seizures, and was otherwise normal, we asked her mother to bring her back during another episode, should one occur.

It was almost a year later when we received a call from Joanne's mother in the middle of the day. "She is doing it again." We didn't remember Joanne, but told her mother to bring her in immediately. A very attractive, dull ten-year-old came into the office. She could answer questions and count, but seemed to be mildly retarded. If her mother had not insisted that this was not Joanne's usual state, and if our records had not confirmed a previously sparkling young lady, we might have been fooled.

An immediate EEG confirmed "spike-wave stupor," a continuous electrical status on the EEG, and after a small dose of diazepam (Valium), she immediately returned to her usual state. When she was admitted from the EEG lab to the ward, the resident wanted to know why we were admitting this perfectly normal, charming young lady. With anticonvulsant medication, she has never had another episode.

There is no evidence that spike-wave stupor causes permanent damage to the brain, even when it goes on for hours or days. However, it clearly disrupts the child's level of function. Spike-wave stupor can easily be treated, but it is far better to prevent these seizures with continued use of an appropriate anticonvulsant medication.

*Although many myths and fears still persist about status epilepticus, with early recognition and appropriate treatment, children who have an episode of status should return to their previous function and have no residual effects.*

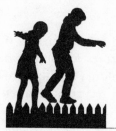

# 11. How Long Do Seizures Need to Be Treated?

Once upon a time it was believed that epilepsy was forever. In those olden days, only fifteen to twenty years ago, physicians were taught never to discontinue anticonvulsant medicine. They were taught not to discontinue the drugs before puberty, because seizures might increase in frequency at puberty, and you were never sure when puberty might start or when it would end. After puberty came driving, and you wouldn't want to stop medication before that, because the child might never be able to get a driver's license. Then physicians were urged not to discontinue medication because the individual was driving. In those days, it was said: "Eventually people will stop taking medicine on their own. Then, if they have a seizure, it will not be the doctor's fault."

NONE OF THOSE OLD TEACHINGS WERE TRUE!

With this old philosophy, many people were kept on medicine for many years, and some are still taking it.

Now we know that:

• Most children outgrow their epilepsy;
• Most children who are free of seizures for two years gradually can be taken off medicine by their physician and will remain seizure-free;
• Many adults do not need to take medicine forever.

Now we know that 75 percent of children who have been free of seizures for four years will remain seizure-free as the medicine is slowly discontinued. Seventy-five percent will also remain free of seizures if they are taken off medicine after being free of seizures for only two years. Now we can even predict which of these children are likely to remain free off medicine and which are likely to have recurrent seizures if the medication is discontinued.

*Remember: Before you begin to worry about having your physician discontinue medication, your child must be seizure-free for at least two years.*

### "What is the chance of my child coming off medicine and staying seizure-free?"

When your child has been free of seizures, on medication, for two years:

- Those children who have had idiopathic seizures, and who have no evidence of neurologic dysfunction, and whose EEG is normal or near normal have a 90 to 95 percent chance of remaining seizure-free without medication;
- Those children who have had epilepsy caused by old and non-progressive brain damage, such as a birth injury or head trauma, have a 40 to 60 percent chance of staying seizure-free off medication, even if their EEGs are moderately abnormal;
- Those children whose EEGs are severely abnormal, and, particularly, if their EEGs are worse than when their seizures began, have a 90 to 95 percent chance of having *more* seizures if medicine is discontinued—even if they have been free of seizures for two years on medicine.

These scenarios represent points on a spectrum. How then does someone decide whether or not medication should be discontinued? or can be discontinued *safely?* Here we have to go back to our risk-benefit analysis (see Chapter 4). Remember that the risks are yours and your child's, as are the benefits. Thus, you both have to be full partners with your physician as these decisions are made.

### "What is the worst that can happen if my child continues taking the medication?"

If your child has been free of seizures for two years and is tolerating his medication well, then probably not much will happen if he continues to take medication. However, if he continues to take medicines for a long time, chronic effects occur that vary with the medicine. In addition, if your child is a girl, eventually she may want to have children. While the risks of any medication on the fetus are small, they are many times greater than no medication at all. If a woman doesn't need medication to control seizures, the baby will be better off not being exposed to these drugs. Also, you'll never know how much better your child will function without medication unless your physician discontinues it.

### *"What is the worst that can happen if we decide to discontinue my child's medicine?"*

Medication should never be stopped suddenly since this could cause status epilepticus. It should only be stopped under your physician's direction. When the medication is decreased slowly, the worst thing that can happen is that your child will have another seizure. The consequences of another seizure vary with the individual's age and circumstances. You and your child will have to determine how much weight to give this matter. When people stop taking medication under their doctor's direction, they tend to worry about having another seizure. In our experience, this concern diminishes over time and is usually negligible after about a year.

### *"What is the best that can happen if my child continues taking the medication?"*

The best that can happen if medication is continued is that your child will be no worse off than he is now. He may also not be as fearful if he is taking medication, even though he is constantly reminded that another seizure may recur. But, unless he takes medication forever, at some time in his life he will need to face this worry. If the decision is to stop medication, you and he should choose the time at which this concern will have the least impact. For example: you might want to discontinue medication at a convenient time during the summer when school is out.

### *"What is the best that can happen if my doctor discontinues my child's medication?"*

The best that can happen is that your child will remain seizure free and that there will be an improvement in his learning and behavior. Many adults say, "I'm not so tired any more. I feel so much better. I can think much more clearly." Many parents say, "Mary is a different child.

Her school work is better. She's not so irritable and she's not so tired all the time. I never realized the medicine was affecting her in that way." Another benefit is that your child would not have to take medication each day, a reminder of his potential problem. He would no longer have "controlled" epilepsy. Now he would be either "recovered" or "cured" and could get on with his life, unimpeded.

For the normal child who has only a 5 to 10 percent chance of having another seizure, we would recommend discontinuing medication. In general, the consequences, should a seizure recur, will be small. For the handicapped child who may have a 50 percent chance of another seizure, we would also recommend trying to discontinue medication. The consequences of another seizure for him are also small, but since he may be less able to compensate for the subtle effects of medication on learning and behavior, the benefits of being free of medication may be even greater. Should a seizure recur, and if it is apparent that the child is functioning better off the original medication, it may be possible to substitute a less toxic anticonvulsant.

*On balance, we believe that avoiding the chronic effects of medication and their effects on learning and psychological function outweigh the risks of another seizure in most children who have been seizure-free for two years.*

### *"Are there any situations where you would discourage someone from discontinuing medicine?"*

Yes. We would recommend continuing medication for the child whose EEG is severely abnormal, where the chance of recurrence is very high, although if the child and parent were determined to try to discontinue medication we would be supportive. In some of the special forms of epilepsy, such as the juvenile myoclonic epilepsy of Janz, or the Lennox-Gastaut syndrome (Chapter 8), where the chance of recurrence of seizures is very high, we would suggest continuing medicine. In each case we would make an individual decision, discuss the risks and benefits of alternative courses of action with the parent and child, and help them to reach a sound decision.

### *"If we stop the medicine, how long will we have to worry about the seizures coming back?"*

Most recurrences happen shortly after the medication is stopped, indeed, many while the medicine is being tapered. One-half of the recurrences happen within six months of stopping medication, 60 to 80 percent occur within one year, and virtually all within two years of stopping the medicine. This is another reason why, if possible, it would be better to discontinue medicine before or during the early teenage years, because the consequence of a seizure would be less severe before the individual has begun to drive or has a job.

*In summary, most epilepsy in children is not forever. Therefore, treatment for most children should not be forever. Decisions about discontinuing medication can begin to be made when the child approaches being seizure-free for two years. You should discuss the risks and benefits of continuing medication and of stopping medication with your physician.*

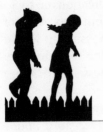

# 12. Other Approaches to Therapy:
## Vitamins, Minerals, and Special Diets

Epilepsy that does not respond to the available anticonvulsants can be enormously frustrating to patients, parents, and physicians. Therefore, it is not surprising that many other approaches to the treatment of seizures have been tried, including the addition of single or multiple vitamins in regular or megadoses to the diet, the addition of varying minerals to the diet, or the adoption of special diets. Although there are abundant testimonials to the benefits of almost everything that has been tried, there is little evidence that most of the claims are justified.

*There is* NO *evidence that epilepsy is caused by a deficiency of vitamins, minerals, or diet.* Having said that, there *are* rare inherited conditions that cause seizures and that will respond to the addition of a vitamin or to dietary manipulation. Could some small portion of other epilepsy cases be a consequence of unknown dietary deficiencies or excesses? It is possible, but that portion must be very small and due to very specific deficiencies. Thus, at the present time, vitamin supplements and special diets (other than the ketogenic diet discussed below) should not replace anticonvulsant therapy.

Despite anecdotal stories, there is no evidence that food allergies or the elimination diets used to control them play any role in the treatment of epilepsy.

## Vitamins

Vitamins are small molecules known to be necessary for certain chemical reactions to take place in the body. Although a balanced diet contains sufficient amounts of vitamins and does not require vitamin supplements, vitamin deficiencies *can* occur when diets are very unusual. Deficiencies also can occur in rare situations where an individual is unable to absorb vitamins from food. There also are very rare inherited conditions in which a person's body chemistry requires unusually large amounts of a specific vitamin. One example of such a rare vitamin deficiency or dependency known to produce epilepsy is deficiency of vitamin B6, or pyridoxine. Lack of B6 may cause difficult-to-control seizures in the newborn. Your physician may give small doses of the vitamin to see whether it controls seizures in these infants. Occasionally, when older children have difficult-to-control seizures, your physician may suggest giving added pyridoxine to see if it is effective.

Except in rare, specific problems, the addition of other vitamins or mineral supplements to a balanced diet is of NO documented benefit in the treatment of seizures.

## Calcium and Magnesium

Calcium is a very important mineral for the normal functioning of brain cells, and low levels of calcium (hypocalcemia) can cause seizures. Hypocalcemia can be a consequence of severe kidney disease when too much calcium escapes from the kidney in the urine. It may also, but rarely, be caused by a hormonal problem that has the same effect. For children with repeated seizures the level of calcium in the blood should be tested. If it is low, then the cause should be sought and extra calcium given if necessary. A deficiency of magnesium, a mineral that interacts with calcium, may cause low blood calcium and, thus, seizures.

## The Ketogenic Diet: Its Risks and Benefits

In the 1920s and early 1930s, phenobarbital and bromides were the only anticonvulsants available to treat seizures. There is an apocryphal story about the young daughter of a New York dentist who had uncontrollable seizures. She was taken to a group of disciples of Bernarr McFadden in Wisconsin, who would pray and fast with individuals for a price. Miraculously, the young lady's seizures ceased. Prayer alone had no effect; prolonged fasting was effective but impractical. Searching for help to find an alternative to fasting, the family interested investigators at Johns Hopkins and elsewhere who were, at the time, studying infant nutrition. These investigators found that when an individual fasts, the body metabolizes its own protein, and large amounts of ketone bodies and uric acid are excreted in the urine. Erroneously believing that this had something to do with seizure control, they found that if the fast was broken by eating protein or carbohydrate, the uric acid disappeared. If the fast was broken with fat, the uric acid excretion continued. A diet was then constructed with minimal protein intake and most of the calories as fat. The diet had virtually no carbohydrates.

The ketogenic diet, named for the ketones excreted in the urine, is one of the oldest forms of therapy for epilepsy. It has fallen into disuse because of the availability of new and effective anticonvulsants. It is far easier to take several anticonvulsant pills each day than to adhere to this rigid and cumbersome diet. However, in situations where modern anticonvulsants are ineffective, or where their side effects are overwhelming, the ketogenic diet often can control seizures completely with few if any side effects on behavior and learning.

The beneficial effects of starvation and dehydration on seizures have been known for centuries. However, starvation and dehydration cannot be maintained over long periods of time. The ketogenic diet was developed to provide the minimal amount of protein necessary for growth, virtually no carbohydrates, and most of the required calories as fat. Numerous studies done in the 1930s found that the diet completely controlled seizures in almost 50 percent of children placed on the regimen and markedly improved seizure control in another 25 percent. However, in the late 1930s, with the introduction of phenytoin (Dilantin) and later other effective anticonvulsants, the ketogenic diet began to be used less frequently. Physicians then became less familiar with its use, and few dieticians were trained to utilize it properly. It is now used only in a few large centers.

At Johns Hopkins, where much of the early work on the diet was performed and where dieticians have continued to be familiar with its use, we have continued to use the diet fifteen or so times each year. A recent review of our results with children placed on the diet only as a last resort—severely handicapped children with frequent seizures refractory to all of the new anticonvulsants—shows that the diet completely controlled seizures in more than half of the cases. Thus, the diet continues to be a very useful form of therapy for properly selected individuals.

The ketogenic diet contains a high ratio of fat to carbohydrate plus protein. Most of the calories are provided as fats, using butter and heavy cream. Seizure control is greatest when the diet contains a ratio of fat calories to protein/carbohydrate calories of 3 or 4:1. A typical meal might consist of a very small portion of meat, fish, poultry, or cheese, a slightly larger portion of fruit, additional fat served as butter or mayonnaise, and a serving of heavy (whipping type) cream. It doesn't sound very palatable, does it? It is this perception of the diet as unappealing that has interfered with its more frequent use.

When your child is severely handicapped by seizures and massive amounts of medication, what do you have to lose by trying the diet? Not much! What do you have to gain? If it works, a lot. If it doesn't, you've lost very little other than the time invested in learning how to prepare the diet. If your child is seizure-free and less drugged, then the rigors of the diet are worthwhile. If the child's seizures continue after one to three months on the diet or if the diet is poorly tolerated, then the diet can be discontinued and the child returned to medication.*

The diet is initiated with several days of starvation and limited fluid intake. The child should be carefully observed during this time for signs of hypoglycemia (low blood sugar)—paleness, sweatiness, unresponsiveness, or seizures. When the child is very ketotic (has a lot of ketones in the urine) and has lost about 10 percent of his body weight, one-third of the diet is begun. The diet is increased over the first two to three days. We usually do this in the hospital since this allows us to instruct the parents in diet preparation. Menus can be selected to fit the child's food preferences. It is surprising how much variety an innovative parent can introduce into this restricted diet.

*WARNING: The diet should not be attempted on your own. The diet will only work when it, and you, are carefully supervised by a dietician familiar with using the diet. The diet may be dangerous if not done properly.*

*WARNING: The diet is deficient in vitamins B and C as well as in calcium and these must be given as supplements in a sugar-free form. Also, remember that today many things like toothpaste, vitamins,*

---

*Although details of the diet are beyond the scope of this book, they may be found in M. Walser, A. Imbembo, S. Margolis, and G. Elfert, *The Johns Hopkins Handbook of Nutritional Management* (Philadelphia: W. B. Saunders Company, 1984).

*and children's antibiotics and cough syrups have added glucose. If your child is on the ketogenic diet, you must read every label carefully and, if in doubt about added sugar, check with your physician, the dietician, or the manufacturer.*

Small deviations in the diet can result in a seizure. Indeed, if a child has been well-controlled on the diet and has a seizure, you can almost be sure that the child has eaten a cookie, a piece of candy, or a bit of dog food. (Yes, small children can get into the dog food!) Should this happen, a day of starvation followed by reinstitution of the diet usually will re-achieve control.

### "Is my child eligible for this diet?"

The diet appears quite effective in children with myoclonic and atonic (drop) types of seizures, the types most resistant to current medications. However, it can be used in virtually all forms of epilepsy. The diet is not used during the first year of life, because the infant is not capable of maintaining the ketosis. There is no upper age limit to its use, but children over the age of four or five who have normal intelligence may have developed sufficient food preferences and sufficient independence that maintaining the diet can be difficult. We have used it successfully in pre-teens and adolescents when the individual and family are well-motivated.

### "Will my child have to remain on this diet for life?"

No. Most children whose seizures are controlled on the diet remain on it for two years. After that time they can gradually be taken off the diet, and the seizures usually do not return, even without additional anticonvulsant drugs.

### "That sounds like a miracle. How does the diet work?"

We don't understand how the diet works. The results do not seem to be merely the effects of the dehydration, or of the ketosis, or of the acidosis (increased amount of acid in the blood) that accompany the diet. We clearly need more research to understand the effects of this diet on seizures.

### "How long will my child have to stay on the diet before we know that it is working?"

Many children with frequent daily seizures will stop having seizures during the starvation phase of the diet. Most for whom the diet will be effective will cease having seizures during the first week. However, since some will respond later, we recommend continuing the diet for one to three months before giving up.

### *"When can we stop the anticonvulsants?"*

If the child is on barbiturates, we often begin to taper them off during the starvation phase, since the barbiturate level may increase and make the child sleepy. We continue the other anticonvulsants until it is apparent that the diet is effective in controlling the seizures and that it is tolerated. Then we slowly taper the other anticonvulsants over several months.

### *"What are the complications of the ketogenic diet?"*

During the starvation phase of the diet, the child's blood sugar may drop, with symptoms like weakness, dizziness, paleness, sweating, and sleepiness. If these occur, it is imperative to measure the blood sugar and to give a small amount of glucose before continuing starvation. We have mentioned that supplementary vitamins and calcium are needed to prevent deficiencies. Your child should gain little weight on the diet if it is properly calculated, and growth may be slightly slowed. However, both will catch up when the diet eventually is discontinued. Despite the high fat content, the diet does not appear to cause atherosclerosis. Kidney stones can occur, but may be prevented by appropriate fluid intake.

### *"Is the diet always a last resort to control seizures?"*

This diet has been used mainly as a last resort. However, since it is so effective when nothing else works, perhaps it should be used earlier in the course of epilepsy, if you and your child are willing to try it as an alternative to medication.

### *"Isn't there any other alternative to the ketogenic diet?"*

There is another form of the diet, called the MCT diet, in which the fats are given in the form of an oil. Although giving fats in this form allows the remainder of the diet to be more flexible, our experience shows that the MCT diet is not as effective as the classic ketogenic diet and that it is less well tolerated. We prefer the standard ketogenic diet.

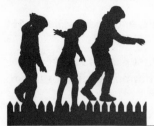

# 13. Surgical Approaches to Epilepsy

❏ Wendy had her first complex partial seizure when she was 13. Her initial evaluation, including a CT scan and EEG, revealed no cause, and medication was prescribed. Phenobarbital made her sleepy, and phenytoin (Dilantin) only slightly reduced the frequency of her seizures, now occurring three to four times a week. Carbamazepine (Tegretol) was added, and the seizures became less frequent. However, Wendy's school work began to suffer while she was taking several medications, and she became depressed. At sixteen she couldn't drive and because of embarrassment she became less social and more isolated. When she was eighteen, valproic acid (Depakene) became available, but despite attempts to adjust medication, her physicians were unable to completely control her seizures. By this time, Wendy's school work had suffered and she had been turned down by the colleges of her choice. She was about to enter the local junior college.

When we first saw Wendy, she was a highly motivated young lady, depressed about the seizures and about her future. She had received psychological counseling, which had helped some, but the seizures—suddenly stopping what she was doing, staring, then wandering about the room, picking at her clothes, and remaining in a confused state for ten to fifteen minutes—were still occurring several times each week despite good levels of medication.

Our evaluation suggested that the seizures came from the right temporal lobe. Surgery was discussed, but Wendy, now twenty-two, was afraid. We worked with her, long distance, to adjust the medications, but she either had problems with drug toxicity or with seizure control. Nevertheless, she finished college and began a masters program in psychology. Finally she decided she was willing to have the surgery. Repeat evaluation suggested that the focus was in the anterior right temporal lobe. This was removed surgically and revealed "mesial temporal sclerosis," an old scar that had not been visible on the scans.

Wendy has had no seizures in the past five years, has finished her Ph.D. in psychology, and says that life and her work are both much easier now without seizures and without any medication. "I only wish that we had done the surgery much earlier," she says. "It would have made growing up so much easier."

❑ Douglas had his first tonic-clonic seizure at 14. The initial CT showed a small abnormality in the anterior left temporal lobe, probably caused by bleeding from abnormal blood vessels. The doctor decided to wait and see what would happen. Six months later Doug began to have complex partial seizures, and he was referred to us. We began administration of carbamazepine (Tegretol) and discussed the option of surgical removal of the malformation both for the control of seizures and because the malformation might bleed again.

The lesion was removed when Douglas was 15, one year after his first seizure. He is now completing high school. He's on the basketball team, and he lives without seizures and without medication.

When we recently asked Doug how he felt about all that had gone on he replied, "It wasn't any big deal. I didn't like having my beautiful hair shaved off, but that's all behind me now."

## Tumor Surgery and Epilepsy Surgery

There are two different reasons to do brain surgery in a patient with seizures. One we call "tumor" surgery, the other "epilepsy" surgery. A "tumor" in the brain may cause seizures. By tumor we mean not only abnormal growths and cancer but also abnormal blood vessels, areas of prior bleeding, and cysts, which may press on the surrounding brain causing seizures. The surgeon or neurologist may recommend removal of the tumor and the seizures may be controlled as well. Removal of these abnormalities is called "tumor" surgery, and its purpose is different from "epilepsy" surgery.

Epilepsy surgery is primarily intended to eliminate the seizures, whether or not a "tumor" is present.

Abnormalities of the brain causing seizures may also be subtle, just local abnormalities of cells or local scarring, with nothing pressing on the surrounding brain. In these cases, separating normal from abnormal ("epileptic") tissue may be more difficult. Removal of these abnormal areas to control seizures is defined as "epilepsy surgery." Sometimes scars, tumors, or blood vessel abnormalities are removed incidentally while removing the abnormal tissue causing the seizures. As we continue our discussion of surgery, we are focusing on epilepsy surgery and not on tumor surgery.

If there is a small, focal area of abnormality in the brain triggering seizures, it would seem far more logical to have that area removed surgically than to take anticonvulsant medication for a lifetime. Thus, surgery *should* be the treatment of choice for partial (focal) seizures if the focus is in a part of the brain that can be safely removed. While logical, this procedure is rarely undertaken. The brain has always been considered a sacred organ, one which should not be violated, and physicians have been reluctant to operate on the brain unless it is absolutely necessary. Patients were, and still are, afraid to have brain surgery. While elective surgery on most other organs is now considered routine, surgery on the brain is still considered by many to be a high-risk and frightening procedure, to be undertaken only as a last resort.

With amazing technological advances that have made it possible to locate a seizure focus in more people with epilepsy and to distinguish normal from abnormal brains, surgery has become far safer. Recent advances have changed our whole approach to children and adults with difficult-to-control seizures. *Still, epilepsy surgery should be considered only when the seizures have not responded to appropriate medications given in appropriate doses and when either the seizures or the medications are* significantly *interfering with the daily life of the patient.*

*Surgery should only be performed after careful evaluation in an epilepsy center with full capabilities for both evaluation and surgery, and then only after careful consideration of the alternatives.*

Three major types of epilepsy surgery are currently performed: "focal excision," which removes the epileptic area thought to be triggering the seizures; "hemispherectomy," or partial hemispherectomy, which removes all or much of one side of the brain when large areas are electrically and functionally abnormal; and "corpus callosum sectioning," an operation cutting the tissue connecting the two hemispheres, thus preventing the spread of the seizures to the other side of the brain. Although modifications of these and other procedures may be devised for specific patients and specific problems, we discuss here only these three more commonly performed procedures. Each is appropriate only for specific seizure problems, and each has its own risks and benefits.

## Surgery for Partial (Focal) Seizures

### General Considerations for Surgery

Partial seizures, or partial seizures that secondarily generalize (Chapter 6) are, by definition, always focal (local) in origin. Any child with partial (focal) seizures deserves some evaluation to find the source of the focal abnormality. If the EEG shows focal slowing or if the child has had several seizures that seem to start from the same area of the brain, then the child should have a CT or MRI scan searching for a focal, structural problem that might require surgery. Surgery is rarely considered in the child who has had only a few seizures unless there is a tumor or vascular abnormality—*rare* causes of seizures in children—and then the surgery done is "tumor" surgery. Douglas, whom we discussed above, was a child with a structural problem who benefited from surgery early in the course of his epilepsy and who was cured by the procedure.

In the absence of a tumor or vascular abnormality, trials of medication are indicated to try to control focal seizures. If the seizures remain persistently focal, then the option of surgery should be considered. Considering the option is not the same as pursuing that option, but whereas only a few years ago surgery was not even contemplated until medication trials had been exhausted, now the new techniques for evaluation, as well as the advances in surgical technique, have made surgery a more reasonable and desirable alternative to lifelong medication, even if that medication controls the seizures.

Consideration for surgery is a multiphased process. It proceeds step-by-step. The process can be stopped at any step if evidence suggests that the child is not a good candidate for surgery.

### Is Your Child a Candidate for Surgery?

The initial step in identifying a candidate for surgery is to question whether your child's focal seizures can be operated on. Do these seizures reliably and repeatedly come from a single area, and can that area be removed safely? These are not questions that you can answer yourself, but questions that your doctor must consider.

We find that the pattern of the clinical seizures is most helpful in the initial screening of who should be a candidate for consideration of surgery. Your child must have a sufficient number of seizures in order to establish a reliable and consistent pattern that can be evaluated. This will take time. If your child's seizures always follow the same pattern (for example, with the seizure always starting in the right hand, or with the head and eyes always turning to the left), this would suggest that the seizures may start in a particular location in the brain. It may also require repeated EEGs to document a consistent area of abnormality.

Routine EEGs may, or may not, show a focal abnormality, and special EEGs may be necessary. If your doctor finds multiple abnormal areas on EEG, then your child is probably *not* a candidate for surgery.

The next question at this stage is whether the focal abnormality, if present, is in an area which can be safely removed. The anterior portions of the frontal or temporal lobes are the portions of the brain that can be removed without causing neurologic problems. Therefore, children whose seizures repeatedly appear to come from these areas should be considered good candidates for evaluation for *possible* surgery early in the course of their epilepsy. If, on the other hand, the seizures appear to come from near the motor or speech area, the likelihood that surgery will cause neurological problems is higher.

Your physician will probably have some thoughts about whether or not your child might be a candidate for surgery. If he has not brought up the subject, it might be appropriate for you to ask him. After your physician has found answers to the two preliminary questions noted above, *and* if your child does seem to be a good candidate, *and* if the seizures are difficult to control with medicines, *then* it is the appropriate time for you and your physician to discuss the possible risks and benefits of surgery. If your child is a good candidate for surgery and you are interested in considering surgery, then the next step in the evaluation can take place.

### Confirming that Your Child Is a Candidate for Surgery

The second step in the process of evaluating your child for surgery should take place in an epilepsy center capable of carrying out the full evaluation *and* the surgery.

If the center does not know your child, they will want to review his records carefully and may want to repeat EEGs and scans before deciding if further evaluation is in order. The center might also think that further trials of medication might be useful before considering further evaluation. Sometimes we find that patients referred to us have pseudoseizures, not true seizures (see Chapter 2). Other children have multiple areas of abnormality and thus are not candidates for surgery. However, if the person is still a possible candidate, then the next step is to document that there is indeed a single seizure focus and that it is in an operable location. This will require video-EEG recording.

Video-EEG monitoring (see Chapter 7) is the use of continuous monitoring of the EEG with simultaneous video recording to document both the clinical and the electrical onset of the seizures. It is essential to appropriate evaluation for surgery. The duration of this monitoring will depend on the center and on the frequency of the seizures. In general, we schedule one week in the monitoring unit, although for an individual with frequent seizures, a few days is often sufficient to analyze enough spells and determine if there is a consistent focus. If the seizures are less frequent, or if they subside in the hospital setting, as they often do, then we may withdraw one or more of the medications to permit seizures to be recorded. Since this drug withdrawal is done in the hospital setting, with trained personnel readily available should status epilepticus occur, the risk of abrupt withdrawal is minimized.

If, after careful analysis of the recorded seizures, a focus is identified, then consideration of surgery can proceed. If the abnormal area is situated far forward in the temporal or frontal lobes, areas that can be safely removed, then it may be possible to proceed directly to surgery. Surgery should never proceed, of course, until you and the surgeon have fully discussed the risks to your child, the chances of controlling the seizures, and any other questions you or your child may have.

### Risk-Benefit Discussion with Your Physicians

Discussion of the possibility of surgery and its risks and benefits should be an ongoing process. Having identified a focus and its location, surgery can become a more serious consideration, and a more detailed discussion of its risks and benefits is possible. The risks will depend on the area to be removed. Surgery is most often performed to remove a focus from the frontal or temporal lobes of the brain, areas from which large amounts of tissue can usually be safely removed without major complications.

As with any operation, there is, of course, a risk of dying or suffering major complications of anesthesia. While the consequences of such a complication could be great, the chances of a major anesthetic complication's occurring are in the range of less than one per one thousand. Infection also is always a risk; so is bleeding or clotting of a blood vessel. All these are potentially serious and capable of causing additional brain damage. Fortunately, these complications occur infrequently.

Generally, as noted, frontal and temporal lobe removals are considered by neurologists and neurosurgeons to be "safe" procedures, but as with any decision-making process, the risks and their magnitude must be weighed against the possible benefits and the chances of those benefits occurring. What are the benefits of the focal operations? The maximum benefit would be freedom from seizures for your child—freedom from taking anticonvulsant medicine and freedom from neurologic deficit due to the surgery. This is everyone's goal. What are the chances of that occurring? Surprisingly, it is difficult to give numerical answers to this question. Surgical centers often quote 60–75 percent "good outcomes." This means that perhaps 50 percent will be cured of their seizures, another 10–25 percent will have substantial decrease in the frequency of their seizures, and about 25 percent—one in four—will not be helped at all.

You cannot, however, apply statistical figures to your child. Your child's chance of success will depend on the cause of the seizures and the exact location of the focus within these lobes. The figures quoted also depend on how a specific center selects its patients for surgery. If they only select "ideal" candidates their success rate will be higher. If they take some of the more difficult patients, they may be less "successful." Your child is unique and, therefore, the discussion and the chances of success are unique. Besides, modern techniques of evaluation may improve your child's chances of having a successful outcome.

Whether the risks of surgery are worth the possible benefits is a very personal decision. The benefits of possibly being totally free of seizures will have different values to different people. The risks each individual and family are willing to take to achieve that condition are also very personal. It is our belief, however, that in general physicians and surgeons have been far too conservative in recommending surgery. Temporal lobe removal may be preferable to taking medication for a lifetime, even if the medication is controlling the seizures with minimal side effects. The anterior part of the temporal lobe on either side, as noted, may be removed without causing neurologic problems. Much of the frontal lobe on either side can also be safely removed.

Because language function is in the more posterior part of the left temporal lobe in most children, surgery that might involve that area requires very careful evaluation in order to weigh the possible risks and benefits. Similarly, since motor function is in the posterior frontal lobe, consideration of surgery near that area also requires careful thought.

## Evaluation of Language

Speech is usually located on the left side of the brain, in the posterior temporal lobe (see Chapter 6). However, in 10 to 15 percent of left-handed people speech is on the right side. It is vital to know where it is before proceeding with surgery.

The Wada test, named after the neurosurgeon Dr. Juhn Wada, is designed to localize speech and memory. A catheter is threaded from the groin of the awake patient up to the internal carotid artery, the main artery supplying one side of the brain. After a small injection of a dye, which can be seen on x-ray, a small amount of barbiturate is injected and that side of the brain is briefly "put to sleep."

As the test begins, the patient is asked to hold his arms up in the air and to count. If the injection is done on the left side of the brain, the right arm becomes weak as the left side of the brain goes "to sleep." If speech is on that same side, the child will simultaneously, but briefly, lose the ability to speak or count. Memory is also tested by showing objects and pictures. When the medication wears off, the patient will be asked to recall the objects he has seen. If lost, speech and memory quickly return when the drug wears off. In this crude fashion the laterality (side) of speech is determined. The same procedure may also be carried out on the other side of the brain, because occasionally speech is located on *both* sides.

If injecting the right side produces no alteration in speech or memory, then it can be assumed that it is safe to operate on that side. If speech is on the left and the surgery is to be done near that area, then far more careful evaluation of speech, language, and the epileptic focus must precede a decision about surgery.

Detailed neuropsychological testing may be performed prior to surgery to assess the person's intellectual function and personality. This may help in understanding if certain parts of the brain previously have been damaged.

## Invasive Studies

When questions about the exact localization of the seizure focus or about the relationship of the focus to important functions such as speech or movement still remain, further studies may be required.

These further studies are "invasive," which means that they require an operation and, therefore, carry some risk. Depth electrodes (wires placed deep in the brain) are used when the focus appears to be deep in the brain and when it is difficult to be certain where seizures are coming from (Fig. 13.1A). Another invasive approach is to "map" the surface of the brain by a plastic sheet (grid) of electrodes placed directly on the surface of the brain (Fig. 13.1B). The grid is utilized when the seizure focus is on the surface of the brain and in areas where other important functions such as speech or motor function might co-exist and could be damaged by the operation. The electrodes in the grid can directly record the abnormal electrical activity from the abnormal area and can be used to stimulate local areas of the brain to assess their function.

While depth electrodes have been used for many years, the use of a grid is relatively new. It is currently used only in very specialized situations. The grid offers a major advance in our ability to define epileptic areas carefully and to separate them from normal tissue. If these procedures are being considered for your child, you should discuss them in detail with the epilepsy center's staff.

## Making the Final Decision

While each step in the process of evaluation of a child for surgery requires careful thought, it is at this point, when all the available information has been collected, that reconsideration of the potential risks and benefits is necessary. We accomplish this with a meeting of the whole team that has been involved in the evaluation. This team includes the epilepsy specialist who has been your child's primary physician, our group of monitoring specialists, those who have carefully assessed language and intellectual function, our counsellor who has been working closely with the child and the family, and the surgeon who will be performing the operation. At this conference we carefully assess where the seizures appear to be coming from, what surgery can be done to eliminate them, what normal functions might be damaged by the surgery, and the risks and the potential benefits of the surgery. At times we decide that, despite all our careful evaluation, surgery should not be performed. After the group reaches consensus, we then present our opinions to the patient and family, who must make their independent decision on whether or not to proceed with surgery, whether their perception of the risks and benefits is similar to ours.

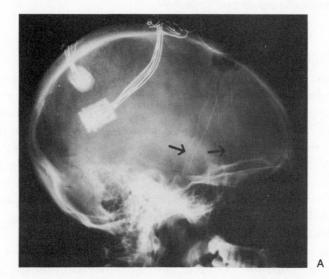

A

**Figure 13.1.** Invasive monitoring. Skull x-ray (A) showing depth electrodes, or thin wires, marked with arrows positioned deep within the brain to record and localize abnormal electrical activity. (B) The thin sheet of plastic with embedded electrodes, shown placed on a model of the brain, is called a grid. The grid is surgically implanted on the surface of the child's brain with wires running to the outside. The electricity is recorded by an EEG machine. The electrodes can also be used for stimulating the underlying brain to localize specific functions.

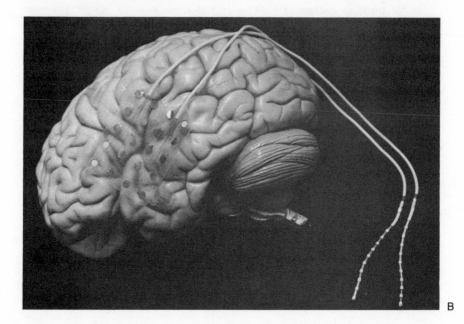

B

## New Noninvasive Research Approaches to Localization

*Positron emission tomography (PET scanning).* Recent technical developments (CT, MRI, grids) have dramatically altered our ability to identify the source of certain children's seizures. Even newer techniques are beginning to improve our ability to study the pathophysiology (the chemical abnormalities) of the seizure areas themselves, rather than just the electrical or anatomic abnormalities. Progress in these areas is awesome.

Positron emission tomography (PET) scanning uses the same principles as CT scanning, but rather than using x-rays as the energy source, derives its images from radioactive particles (positrons), derived from chemicals injected into the body that reach the brain. Thus it is now possible to study, for example, how parts of the brain use glucose (sugar) by giving the body a form of glucose with the radioactive label. The portion of the brain actively using the glucose takes up more of the radioactivity and looks different in the picture produced. We are beginning to be able to study other chemicals and neurotransmitters associated with epilepsy. Positron emission tomography is a research technique we hope will eventually become useful in the clinical management of children with seizures.

*Single photon emission computerized tomography (SPECT scanning).* SPECT scanning, a variation of PET scanning, is less expensive and requires less equipment, but, at present, is far less precise in defining the abnormal area. However, since it is far faster than a PET scan, it may ultimately be better for identifying the changes that occur during a brief seizure. As the equipment improves, SPECT may become more useful and more widely available.

*Magnetic resonance spectroscopy.* Magnetic resonance imaging, which we have previously discussed as a technique for visualizing brain structures, can also be used in a somewhat different form to study brain metabolism. Used in this fashion it is called magnetic resonance spectroscopy. By using far more powerful magnets and different receivers, this technique can "tune in" to the energy changes that occur as one chemical compound is converted to another within the living cells. Thus, as energy is utilized to fire cells during seizures, this energy can be detected and analyzed. As cell membranes change with this firing, or with recovery after their electrical discharge, these changes can be studied. As this new technology continues to develop, it should be possible to understand better the chemistry and spread of human seizures and to develop and visualize the effects of new drugs to block the development and spread of seizures.

*Magneto-encephalography.* If the U.S. Navy can use changes in magnetic fields to detect a submarine 1,000 feet under the sea from a satellite many thousands of feet in the air, then we should be able to detect the changes in magnetic fields generated by a seizure focus two inches under the scalp. And we are beginning to do so.

Submarines, being made of metal, create a minute disturbance of the earth's magnetic field, a disturbance that can be accurately localized by the proper instrumentation in the satellite. Using similar technology, laboratory investigators are beginning to be able to localize the tiny changes in magnetic fields of the surrounding brain, created by the firing of cells. In not too many years it should be possible to localize accurately epileptic foci deep within the brain.

Progress in these areas is mind-boggling.

## Surgery for Other Types of Seizures

### Hemispherectomy

Sometimes the seizure activity, while lateralized to one side of the brain, is not sufficiently localized for removal of only a small focal area. More extensive surgery may be both necessary and helpful. Sometimes we have to take out extensive amounts of the brain or even one half of the brain, hemispherectomy.

Yes, it is possible to remove one half of the brain and still have a child of normal intelligence whose only disabilities are difficulty using the arm on the opposite side and a hemianopsia, meaning that he can't see off to that side of his body. Such children are able to go to regular schools. When older, they can hold full-time jobs and live virtually normal, independent lives. Hemispherectomy is rarely performed, only perhaps ten to twenty times a year in this country. It is mentioned here so that you will know that it does exist and that in very carefully selected situations—when the child has severe damage to only one side of the brain, and already has damage to motor function on the other side of the body, and experiences uncontrollable seizures—a heroic operation such as this can be done. It can be life-saving and allow an otherwise profoundly handicapped child to lead a far more normal life, one free of seizures.

Rarely, or so it seems, a child is born with major abnormalities on only one side of the brain or sustains damage or inflammation (Rasmussen's syndrome [see Chapter 8]) to just one hemisphere of the brain. If your child's seizures are consistently coming from one side of the brain and do not respond to medication, it may be worth discussing the possibility of hemispherectomy with your physician.

Hemispherectomy is not a procedure for everyone, not even for everyone with damage to one side of the brain. It is major surgery that should only be done in a small number of epilepsy centers with experience with the procedure. The outcome for the child depends primarily on the normality of the remaining hemisphere. Indeed, it seems from these children that *no* brain tissue on one side is preferable to the constant electrical interference coming from abnormal brain tissue. It appears that this constant electrical interference impairs the function of the good side. Beth is a good example.

❏ **Beth was a bright, vivacious, almost five-year-old when she fell off of a see-saw and had a generalized seizure. A CT scan showed atrophy in the left hemisphere, but she had no neurological deficit. Shortly thereafter she began to have more seizures on the right side of her body. They did not respond to medication, and gradually she began to limp on the right leg and to have increasing difficulty with speech. Clearly something was continuing to happen to the left side of her brain. Another hospital diagnosed Rasmussen's syndrome and said there was nothing they could do, that this viral-like process would continue to destroy her brain.**

**Six months later her seizures were occurring several times a day and her speech and right-sided paralysis had worsened. She was seen at Johns Hopkins, where we agreed that she had Rasmussen's syndrome. We told the family that this condition would inevitably become worse, that children with it become retarded and severely handicapped. We said that this progression would occur over several years. We told them that the only treatment was to remove the left side of Beth's brain.**

**Since at this time Beth was walking, talking, and had only slight intellectual deterioration, the family, quite understandably, was reluctant to subject their daughter to a risky operation that would leave her paralyzed on one side and might cause a problem with her ability to speak. They decided to wait.**

**Six months later, when Beth was clearly having more difficulty with her seizures, with the right side of her body, and with school, they decided to have the operation.**

**The operation was a success! After a stormy post-operative period, Beth has made a remarkable recovery. She is left-handed and uses her right hand only minimally. Her speech and reading are entirely normal. She has had no seizures since surgery and is on no medications. She is now in the regular third grade, doing well, keeping up with her classmates, telling "knock-knock" jokes, and learning how to play soccer. Clearly for Beth, half a brain is far better than a badly functioning whole brain.**

The choice is not always between removing a small part of one side of the brain and removing an entire hemisphere. These are the two extremes. Large parts of one side of the brain can, when appropriate, be removed. The risks and benefits of these operations depend on the abnormality causing the seizures and the area of the brain to be removed.

### Sectioning of the Corpus Callosum

The corpus callosum is the major pathway connecting one hemisphere of the brain with the other. Some seizures that are focal or multifocal in origin will spread throughout the cortex by the pathway of the corpus callosum to become generalized tonic-clonic seizures. Others will spread by this pathway to deeper structures and lead to atonic and minor-motor drop spells. When an individual is severely handicapped by these generalized seizures, and when the seizures are unresponsive to anticonvulsant medication, sectioning of the corpus callosum may prevent spread of the seizure and abolish the generalized component. Sectioning (cutting) of the corpus callosum does not stop focal seizures, and indeed may sometimes increase them, but focal seizures are more easily tolerated than generalized ones.

After this operation, often done in two stages, there is usually a 50 to 70 percent decrease in the atonic and generalized tonic-clonic seizures. There is little experience with this procedure in young children, where its success rate and its effect on the child's developing nervous system are less understood.

This operation seems to be gaining support as more procedures are performed and the results better defined. Unlike the hemispherectomy patients, who seem to make important gains in intellectual function after surgery and sometimes improvement in their motor function as well, after corpus callosum section, children and adults seem less likely to experience substantial intellectual or motor improvement. The life of these individuals may be dramatically improved, however, with cessation of the akinetic seizures.

*Surgery can sometimes provide "the answer" to seizures that are not controllable with medication and it can sometimes "cure" seizures that are focal or one-sided. Surgery is always worth considering.*

*But considering surgery is a multi-step process that requires careful evaluation at each step. Surgery itself is only the final step in the decision-making process.*

# Part Four

# Coping with Epilepsy

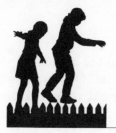

# 14. Coping with Seizures and Epilepsy

There are many different kinds of seizures, and each may affect you and your child in a different fashion. Some children will have only one seizure. Others may have many. You, the parent, will have to find a way of coping, and so will your child. The child's strategy will vary with his or her age, and the strategies of both of you will vary with your personalities as well as with the type and frequency of seizures. But common themes run through all these variations.

Since a single seizure usually has its greatest effect on the parent, it is parents of these children who need advice first. In the second part of this chapter, we discuss how parents and a child can cope with epilepsy itself.

## The First "Big" Seizure

### What You Should Know

*"Richard just had a seizure!" you shouted at your husband over the phone. "He's on his way to the emergency room in an ambulance! They said that he had a grand mal seizure! Meet me there right away!"*

A generalized tonic-clonic, shaking seizure (once called grand mal) is the type most frightening to parents. This one seizure has changed your life. Can you ever look at your child the same way again? Can you really let him go out and play in the backyard without watching him? Suppose he has another seizure? Maybe he could hurt himself. What would the neighbors think if they knew? Will your best friend still let her son come over to play? Will she take the responsibility of watching him? How about the school? Do you want them to know? Do you want it on his records? Will the school allow him to be normal, to do all the things his classmates are doing?

The first thing you need is information. You need to talk to your doctor about what he thinks caused the seizure, about tests and treatment, and about your child's future. If your child's seizure was related to infection or head trauma (a provoked seizure), it is unlikely to recur. When your child recovers and whatever caused the seizure is gone, the seizures will be gone. If the seizure was caused by a fever (a febrile seizure), your child will probably need a few tests, but no treatment, and your child will outgrow these seizures as he gets older.

But in more than half of the cases of seizures in childhood, no cause can be found. If no cause is discovered, that is, if your child has had an idiopathic seizure, the chance of recurrence is about 30 percent. In this situation, where you don't know the future, it's understandable that your anxiety may be higher. We emphasize to worried parents that the best thing is *not* to be able to find a cause because seizures of unknown cause are most likely to be controlled with medication and most likely to be outgrown, even if they recur. The causes we find are usually worse than the causes that we can't find. This seems difficult for parents to believe. But it's the truth.

Even if the doctor finds a cause for the seizure—a scar, a tangle of blood vessels, or even a tumor—usually something can be done, as discussed earlier, or at least you know the cause and can focus your anxiety.

### "Will my child be retarded?"

No! A single tonic-clonic seizure does not cause mental retardation or brain damage! Nor do recurrent seizures cause mental retardation or brain damage. It is true that tonic-clonic and other seizures occur more often among children who already have brain damage, learning problems, or mental retardation, but there is no evidence that seizures make these conditions worse. *Most* children with such problems do not have seizures, and *most* children who have seizures do not have these problems.

Of course you are afraid that seizures will recur. But don't let this anxiety control your life or your child's life. Don't allow it to make you so overprotective that your child can't play or go outside without your

constant supervision. If no new seizure comes, think of the single seizure like a fall out of a tree, something frightening at the time but over
and not influencing your life or your child's life forever.

If seizures do recur, most likely they will recur within two to three
months after the first seizure. It might be reasonable to be a bit more
cautious during this brief period. Maybe your child shouldn't be climbing trees or be in other potentially dangerous situations during this
time. But there's no reason why he can't swim, play most sports, go on
field trips, and lead an otherwise normal life.

### What Do You Tell Your Child?

Be truthful and be simple. What you should tell your child depends
on your child's age, sophistication, and level of understanding. It is best
to be truthful. Otherwise, sooner or later you may get trapped in a web
of lies and cover-ups that will only make things worse. If your child does
not ask questions, it may be because he's too frightened or unable to
articulate his fear. So don't take his silence as meaning he has no
concerns. Remember that your child probably has no memory of the
event that was so frightening to you. His first memory is likely to be of
awakening in the ambulance or in the hospital emergency room. He is
likely to be frightened because he doesn't know what happened—and
is as fearful now of the unknown as you were.

To a young child, your explanation may be as simple as, "You had a
seizure. You couldn't talk to me for a few minutes, and Mommy and
Daddy got very excited and called the doctor, but he says that you're
fine."

For an older child, you might talk about what a seizure is, about
electricity in the brain, and tell him that a seizure is like a short circuit or
a little static on the radio. The pre-teenager or teenager needs a more in-
depth explanation. Your doctor or a nurse should do this, but you
should discuss it with your child as well. He has heard about seizures
and may have many misunderstandings. Give your child a chance to ask
questions. Get him some of the Epilepsy Foundation's publications.

Explain that while there is no guarantee that a similar episode will
not recur, most children never have another one. He is still your normal
boy (or girl) and everything is fine now. Be truthful and reassuring. Let
him know that you were scared, too, but that when you understood
what had happened you were not afraid.

### What Do You Tell Other Children?

Using the same criteria we've discussed above about age appropriateness, reassure your other children. Brothers and sisters need to understand what happened, why you're upset, why you may be treating their brother or sister differently, and whether it will ever happen to them (see Chapter 18). Friends and playmates or schoolmates may or may not need to know depending on whether they witnessed the seizure. If they did, you obviously need to explain. You need to reassure them that their friend is all right and that they can't catch a seizure as if it were a cold. If friends didn't see the seizure happen, you should consider the pros and cons of telling them about something that may never happen again. Remember that your child may tell them something on his own.

### What Do You Tell Grandparents and Friends?

What you tell grandparents and friends depends on many factors. There is no right answer. After a single seizure in a child who is otherwise well, you might decide to tell them nothing. Or you might decide to give them the same frank, simple explanation that you give to older children. The most frightening thing about seizures is the uncertainty. At this stage no one knows if or when they will occur. This frightening anticipation of the unknown is often far worse than the reality of a second seizure itself.

There is something to be gained and something to be lost by discussing the seizure with family and friends. Saying nothing may prevent some over-protection and constant observation. But informing them about the seizure may allow them to cope better should another seizure occur. Reassurance to grandparents and friends that seizures are common, benign, non-life threatening, and do not indicate a brain tumor or any other bad disease of the brain, may be an important ingredient in helping your child lead a normal life.

What you tell others depends on who the others are, their relationships to you and your child, and the frequency of their contact—and their personalities. You will have to use your own judgment, but, in general, we prefer openness.

### What Do You Tell the School?

In the best of all possible worlds, clearly you should tell the school about the seizure. Unfortunately, this is not the best of worlds. Prejudice, misconceptions, overconcern, and fear of seizures still exist. Therefore, there is no simple correct answer to the question. In general, there is no need to tell the school about a single seizure. There is nothing school officials can do, or should do, about your child. They need not watch him more carefully unless he is participating in gymnastics that would place him at heights or is swimming unsupervised. They should not restrict him from playing on sports teams or at recess. He should be allowed to go on field trips and to do everything the other children do. Since there is nothing special school personnel need to do after a single seizure, it's probably not necessary to let them know about it. What or whether you tell the school about the seizure may depend on your assessment of the teacher, the principal, and the school nurse and how you think they will react to the information. If your son or daughter does have another seizure, and if it occurs in school, you will wish that you had told them if you did not. After a second or third tonic-clonic seizure, or with epilepsy, it's a different matter, to be discussed later.

This same philosophy applies to day care and to babysitters. Individuals acting as surrogate parents should have the same information and philosophy about overprotection as you have.

## Recurrent Tonic-Clonic Seizures: Epilepsy

If seizures do recur a parent may use different coping mechanisms than a child. You have already been through the initial shock of seeing tonic-clonic shaking. You have probably come to terms with your initial anxiety. Perhaps you know what to do this second time and are less frightened than at first. But you may be discouraged. Your hopes that a seizure would not recur have been dashed. What is worse, your physician has now used the word "epilepsy." Although epilepsy simply means recurrent seizures, the term carries yet a lot of baggage—myths, mystiques, and prejudices, as we have discussed earlier in this book.

When many people think of epilepsy, they think of the child who is severely handicapped by continuing seizures. Yet they are a small subgroup of children with epilepsy. The largest group are those with "benign epilepsy of childhood," which seems to be outgrown, and a third group has seizures that can be controlled with medicines and that also are, often, outgrown. For most children (eight out of ten) with epilepsy, seizures can be controlled—yes, completely controlled. When a child's epilepsy is under control, it shouldn't significantly alter his life or yours. The myths are wrong!

For one in five children with epilepsy, however, seizures may be difficult to control. Control will require trying out different medications, coping with their side effects, and perhaps even surgery. Your life and your child's life are obviously going to change in significant ways.

Which group will your child fit into? After just a second, or even after a third tonic-clonic seizure, it may be difficult to tell.

### "Benign" Epilepsy of Childhood

Once upon a time epilepsy was considered a chronic disease. People who had two or more seizures had epilepsy, and it was believed that they were doomed to seizures forever.

Now it is recognized that:

• 70 percent of children whose seizures are controlled for two years can go off medication and remain seizure-free. These children have either outgrown their epilepsy or have been "cured";
• One in five children who have one tonic-clonic seizure and a normal EEG will have a second seizure, whether or not they are treated;
• Children who are otherwise normal, who have no evidence of prior damage or dysfunction of the brain, are likely to outgrow their epilepsy.

Benign epilepsy of childhood is a new concept, one not universally accepted, but one we are convinced by observation really exists. Our conviction is reinforced by the fact that the threshold for seizures increases as the young child's brain matures and is more resistant to seizures, and also by the fact that genetic tendencies toward seizures are influenced by age—most children "outgrow" their epilepsy, whether treated or not.

How do you know if your child has benign epilepsy of childhood? After a second seizure neither you nor your doctor can be sure, but, if your child is neurologically and intellectually normal and if the EEG (brain wave test) does not show a lot of abnormalities, then there is good reason to hope. Only time will tell.

## Controlled Epilepsy of Childhood

Even if your child has a number of seizures, and even if it is difficult to find the best medicine to control them, there is still a substantial chance that they will be controlled. There is also a very good chance that after they are controlled for two years, medicine can be discontinued. Your child will have outgrown his seizures. The seizures of 80 percent of children will be controlled, and most of those children will cease taking medication. Thus, most children will not have epilepsy forever.

Even with these encouraging thoughts, when your child has had recurrent seizures, many emotions come into play. It is not uncommon for a person to vacillate between fears, grieving, and anger. The first emotion most people experience is fear.

## Coming to Terms with Epilepsy: Fear, Grieving, Anger, Acceptance

Fear is parents' *normal* response to hearing that their child has epilepsy. It is really fear of the unknown. Information helps make the unknown known. Reality is always less frightening than what you imagine.

Grieving is another emotion that parents must go through when faced with epilepsy. You are sad and grieve for the child whom you think no longer exists as before. You grieve because of your concerns about what epilepsy might do. You grieve for yourself because you're embarrassed and fearful. You grieve because the seizures may present difficulties. You will now have to take time to go to the doctor; it will interfere with your job, your activities, your interests. All of these feelings are common and normal. Indeed, we worry about the parent who shows no signs of grieving. You have to go through grief before you can achieve acceptance.

How do you cope with this grief? It's all right to cry, to feel sorry for yourself and your child. You need to realize that you may not be able to cope all alone. Grieving is much easier when it is shared with someone else. Another person can help you put your grief in perspective. You need to reach out and find support. You may find this within your own home by talking about your fears and concerns with a member of the family. You may find it from another parent or group of parents. The Epilepsy Foundation of America or your local affiliate may be able to put you in touch with resources that will help you deal with these feelings. While grieving is a normal stage, it has to come to an end and ultimately be replaced by a more productive approach to living with epilepsy.

Anger is often the next stage. You're angry at your child for having done that terrible thing, even though you know the seizure was not his fault and that your anger is irrational. You're angry because the ambulance took so long to come, angry that the emergency room was so crowded and inefficient, angry that the nurse was not more considerate, and angry that the doctor didn't take more time examining your child and explaining things to you. You are angry at the system and the world, at your husband (or wife) because he or she is not more concerned or involved or is too concerned and involved, angry at yourself for being angry.

Again, all these reactions are perfectly normal. Different people handle them differently and at different rates. Your husband (or wife) may be at a different stage than you. He or she may be more fearful and not yet have progressed to the stage of grieving or anger. Occasionally a person moves through these stages rapidly, but more often it takes weeks and sometimes months; eventually you will get through them. You can deal with anger in many of the same ways you managed to deal with grief. Talking to others may help you to put your anger in perspective. Communication between parents can be difficult; your husband or wife may not understand your feelings. You may resent a seeming insensitivity. Openness and communication are the only way to deal with these feelings of anger. You may need someone to help you find a way to talk about it with your spouse.

Anger is often long lasting, but can be made productive. If you're angry at the school because of their attitude toward your child, perhaps the best way to handle it is to educate the school system so that they may treat the next child better. If you're angry at your doctor, it may be important to discuss with him why you are angry. Discuss what he said, or what he didn't say, that made you upset. Sometimes your doctor may have said things that were inappropriate, but often you have misunderstood what he said or what he meant to say. Communications are always difficult, particularly in times of stress. Talking should improve matters.

Anger, of itself, is not productive. A person who continues to be angry ultimately alienates those who could be supportive.

Acceptance takes time. It, too, has many different stages. We would like to suggest the power of positive thinking and will discuss it more extensively in Chapter 15. Some parents would like to deny that a seizure ever occurred. These parents might say, "It won't happen again, and I won't let the seizure affect my life or my child's life." But it did occur, and it may recur, and it did affect your life. Whatever approach you take, and different individuals take different approaches, all of these phases should eventually lead to acceptance.

Acceptance means that you can consider your child a normal child who happens to have seizures. It means realizing that your child is not an "epileptic." Lack of acceptance, by comparison, can lead to over-protection, over-permissiveness, lack of discipline, and an inability to set limits for your child.

❑ Butch was sixteen when he came to us. Butch had had three generalized tonic-clonic seizures in the previous several years. He had been taking phenobarbital and had recently had a fourth seizure. Butch had given up football and was barely passing in school. The family told us that they just couldn't control him. He was staying out late with his friends, drinking beer, and they suspected that he was experimenting with drugs. They asked us if there wasn't some medication that would control his seizures so they could get their old Butch back.

As we talked with his parents, it was apparent that the seizures and medication were only minor issues. His behavior problems were partly related to Butch's feelings about himself and his seizures. But epilepsy had paralyzed his family. They felt so sorry for Butch because of the seizures that they could not bring themselves to put normal restrictions on him. They were unable to set limits on his behavior. They overcompensated for what they saw as a major disability. Butch was far more handicapped by the lack of discipline, an important element of good parenting, than he was by his seizures.

We were able to help Butch's parents realize how their attitudes, although well intentioned, were handicapping Butch. Butch had taken control of the family and was neither ready for that control nor comfortable with it. He had gone so far that he was also manipulating the medical situation. He refused to let us draw routine blood work that would have been necessary in changing to a more appropriate medication—one that might have had less impact on his behavior. Counselling took weeks, but eventually we were able to develop a contract with Butch. We helped his parents to set limits. We helped him to focus

**on the possibility of driving, a much desired goal. We enabled him to be a participant in the control of his epilepsy and his life, so that neither he nor epilepsy were the dominant force in his family.**

**It was the overcompensation by his loving family that had led to this intolerable situation and handicapped Butch.**

When your child has had only one seizure and has recovered, it is hard to accept the truth that he is unchanged, that he's no different from the child he was before the seizure. It will take time to accept the fact that the seizure is in the past, that the world has not collapsed, that your child is not retarded or brain-damaged. Indeed, he probably has forgotten anything ever happened. It will take time for you to accept the fact that your child *can* go out and play, *can* go to the neighbor's house, *can* go on camping trips.

When your child has had recurrent seizures, epilepsy, it is even more difficult to realize that often very little has changed. Since most seizures can be controlled, children can return to their normal lives and, in an important sense, nothing need change. Children, of whatever age, still require the same love, attention, limits, and goals.

But in a different sense everything has changed. Your child has to take medicine, at least for a time, and is reminded, at least for a time, that a seizure could happen again. He feels different and may be treated differently by teachers and classmates. He may have some side effects from the medications that he is taking, or he may think that an ordinary upset stomach or school problem is caused by his epilepsy or medication. Both you and your child must find a way to accept the situation. Acceptance may come quickly if seizures are brought under control. Acceptance comes when you realize that you can't change the past and that the future holds many options.

## Helping Your Child Cope with Epilepsy

Your child will go through the same emotional stages you have faced. The manifestations of these stages will vary with the child's age and maturity and with the kinds of seizures.

Fear is real for many of these children. Children may fear dying even though they have no concept of death. This fear of dying should be dealt with forthrightly. All people fear losing control and the fact that one of these seizures could happen at any time. Educating your child about what actually happens during his seizures, what they look like to others, and that he always returns to his previous normal state may help him to adjust to this fear. For the older child, the fear of embarrassment may be even worse than the fear of death. "What will my friends think of me? Suppose I wet myself? Suppose this happens at a dance or in school?" Acceptance by one's peers is critical in adolescence. The worst thing that can happen is that somebody will notice that he is different.

Helping your child to understand epilepsy and accept it to the point where he can explain it to his friends and classmates is the most important element in overcoming these fears.

❏ **Judy told us that seizures had ruined her life. She felt she no longer had friends. She had given up field hockey because she was afraid that a seizure might happen on the field. She now hated school. Even though her seizures had come under control, she was an unhappy young lady. We finally got her to begin to accept her epilepsy by encouraging her to tell the field hockey coach that she had seizures and that they were controlled. Getting her to go back out for the team was the first step in rebuilding her life. Since she could play with the team, she began to realize that she wasn't different from her teammates. As she felt better about herself, her school work improved and her attitude shifted. When she was able to tell classmates about the seizures and what it was like to feel different, Judy began to realize that the rest of the kids never really felt she was different. She realized that her isolation was self-imposed because she was worried that they *might* feel that she was different. The problem was within her and not them. Judy had regained her self-esteem.**

Grieving also occurs in children. Initially the older child or adolescent will think that life has ended, that he can no longer do the same things other children are doing. If you impose unwarranted restrictions, this may be self-fulfilling. This is one of the reasons why it is so important that your child be allowed to participate to the fullest extent possible. Even when restrictions are needed because of the frequency or severity of the seizures, it is important that you find activities in which your child can participate and achieve safely. These are very important ingredients in helping your child develop self-esteem.

Here are a few examples of how children can be helped through these stages:

❏ **Melissa is still grieving. This bright, articulate, theatrical teenager has had staring spells for almost nine months. Although she had been to many** doctors, we were the ones who finally told her that she had epilepsy. Even though she has now begun to take her medicine reliably and has had no seizures in two months, she feels sad. Seizures no longer interfere with any of her multiple activities. There are no side effects from medication. But she feels different, and she is still angry. We have helped her move toward acceptance by offering her an opportunity to meet with other young people who have seizures, youngsters who have already been through some of these stages. We can already see a difference—a willingness to channel these feelings in a productive way. We see a young lady who is beginning to believe that she is not handicapped by her seizures.

☐ Sean still feels sad. Although only nine, he coped with his seizures by talking about them incessantly to all his classmates and friends. Unfortunately this was not productive and resulted in negative reaction. Most children didn't care and so they ignored him, or they were angry at him for bothering them. Understanding that there are lots of people who have seizures had a profound impact on him. We simply told him that we could fill the Orioles' baseball stadium with people from Maryland who have epilepsy. And finally, meeting another child with epilepsy who understood his feelings has made it possible for him to begin to put his seizures into perspective. He no longer feels alone.

Both of these children were grieving and had not accepted their epilepsy. Melissa had internalized the problem and withdrawn, while Sean had externalized his difficulties and was making himself a nuisance. Neither response was productive.

Children, like adults, ultimately need to accept their epilepsy if they are to be happy and productive citizens. They need to realize that epilepsy is only one part of their life, and for most not the dominant part. People should be defined by the kind of person they are, not a condition they have.

Perhaps most important to a child's acceptance of epilepsy is a feeling of self-esteem. For any child to achieve his full potential, he must feel good about himself and able to achieve.

One aspect of self-esteem is a child's feeling of control over his epilepsy and his life. This is why the child should participate in his treatment. Certainly the older child must know why he is taking medicine. A parent who tells his child that he's taking medication because, "It's good for you" or "It's a vitamin and will make you stronger" has not accepted his child's epilepsy and is not allowing the child to accept it either. Also, we encourage parents to let the child, from almost any age, be responsible for taking his own medication. The younger child will require supervision. The older child and adolescent can supervise himself, or learn to, and, in doing so, control and "own" his epilepsy. It is a first step toward achieving control and ownership of his life.

An individual is known by what he can do, not by what he can't do. If you focus on your child's limitations and wish for things that are not realistic, your child is likely to become a failure in your eyes and in his own and fail to achieve his potential. Recognizing your child's potential for achievement is a first step in helping him to recognize his own capabilities. Rewarding achievement is far more productive than focusing on failure.

### What Do You Tell Grandparents and Your Friends?

When your child has had a second or third seizure, family and friends need to be informed. Your child has probably been started on medication and could experience side effects or even temporary changes in personality from the medication. The likelihood of your child having a further seizure is now high enough that family and friends should be informed. They should know what these "frightening episodes" look like and what they should do if another occurs. They should know about the various false myths about epilepsy. Most of the time your child will be normal. Make sure epilepsy is not blown out of proportion. Don't let your friends and relatives dwell on it. If they understand, perhaps they can avoid the overprotection and restrictions that deprive your child of normal experiences.

### What Do You Tell the School and His Classmates?

Teachers are an important part of your child's environment and can be enormously helpful to the child with epilepsy. If they are informed and properly educated, the teacher will know what to do and what to say to classmates should a seizure occur in school. They need to be prepared should a tonic-clonic seizure occur. They can be very helpful in alerting the parent and physician to changes in performance or personality that might be related to drug toxicity.

One of the prevailing myths is that children with epilepsy are stupid or have learning problems. According to many studies, children with epilepsy do tend to have more difficulties in school, but this may be a consequence of fear or anxiety, his own and others'. Nor does this mean that all children with epilepsy have learning problems. Most children with epilepsy do not. Some teachers may see learning problems that aren't there. They may be responding to the myths. But often, the teacher is sensitive to your child's needs. If she points out problems, your physician can evaluate whether they are related to medication. The school may be able to devise an individual educational program to meet your child's needs, if one is required.

Learning problems may not be the result of epilepsy at all. Many children who never had epilepsy don't learn easily. Or, as noted, problems may be a side effect of medication. A change in your child's personality or in his abilities when medication is started may signal such a cause. Early identification of this possibility may allow the physician either to reduce the dose of the drug or to change the medication (see Chapter 19).

To be sure that teachers, school nurses, and principals have accurate information, you may provide some of the excellent pamphlets available either directly from the Epilepsy Foundation of America or from a local affiliate. Many pamphlets are written so that a young child can understand them and are available either free or for only a nominal charge. Pamphlets such as *Because You Are My Friend* explain epilepsy in simple terms to a young child's siblings and friends and, when appropriate, can be used in the child's classroom. Your local epilepsy association can probably provide speakers or perhaps the wonderful puppet show "Kids on the Block," and will try to help educate the school. A brief classroom session may help your child's classmates be more understanding, helpful, and friendly should they see your child have a seizure.

## Absence Seizures

If your child has staring spells or absence seizures—instances where he or she briefly stops and stares, perhaps with some smacking of his lips, picking at his clothes, or confusion—the chances are that he or she has not had just a single episode. These brief spells are usually diagnosed only after many have occurred. Since you first recognize the problem after the fifth, the tenth, or the one hundredth spell, it is obvious that they are likely to continue to recur unless treated with medication.

While less frightening than the tonic-clonic seizure, staring spells cause a particular type of anxiety. Parents are worried that they won't

even know when their child is having a seizure. "Is Jane just daydreaming like all children do, or is she having an absence seizure?" "Should I
have yelled at Billy for not taking out the garbage? Did he not hear me?
Did he disobey? Or was he having an absence seizure?" Since these
seizures are brief and subtle and, therefore, difficult to recognize, it is
probably even more important to tell neighbors, friends, grandparents,
and the school about the spells. This awareness will permit other people
to notice when they occur, to be more tolerant of "daydreaming," and
to be a bit more careful when the child is crossing the street or in a
situation where loss of awareness could cause harm. Also, because this
type of seizure is likely to occur far more frequently than tonic-clonic
seizures (sometimes many times each day or several times per week),
staring spells are more likely than the single tonic-clonic seizure to
interfere with the child's functioning.

Again, it is important to be truthful, but since the child will be
unaware of these spells unless someone tells him, the explanation needs
to be handled with sensitivity. "You have little blackouts, episodes where
you don't know what is going on. They're like static on the radio, a brief
second or two when you can't hear the music." It is important to use
terms appropriate for the age and understanding of the child and to make
sure that the words you use are not frightening. Better for you to tell him
than for him to be asked awkward questions or be told disturbing stories
by other children.

You need to give your child the opportunity to let you know he's
missing things in school—for example, instructions or the end of a
story. We know of one child who assumed that life was just a series of
blank spaces. His class was making a movie about a train going by, and
he wanted to cut out frames of the film. When asked why, he told his
teacher that's how he saw it—with short blank spots between the pictures. It was then that his teacher became aware that there were frequent, very brief, gaps in his attention and that the diagnosis of absence
seizures was eventually made.

These simple absence seizures can usually be brought completely
under control with medication, although it may take several weeks to
gain control. Until then, the child's activities should be more carefully
supervised, with caution and concern but without over-protectiveness
or panic.

Teachers are a very important, perhaps even crucial part of the evaluation and treatment of a child who has absence seizures. There are few other times when a child is consistently under observation and when brief lapses in attention can be readily recognized. It is not uncommon for the teacher to be the first to recognize these lapses of attention. Some parents feel guilty because they did not notice these lapses themselves, but in the structured atmosphere of the classroom, they are often easier to see and recognize than in the more informal atmosphere of a family. And once they are recognized the teacher can be your child's best ally by noting spells and possible side effects of medication.

On the other hand, because of the myths about epilepsy, an uninformed or biased teacher may now treat your child as if he has a learning problem or is dumb. Normal daydreaming may be misperceived as staring spells. A child who is daydreaming may or may not respond if called, but will certainly respond if the teacher goes over and touches him. When a child does not respond he is more likely to be experiencing absence seizures.

## Complex Partial Seizures

In complex partial seizures, as with absence seizures, the child stops, stares, and is unaware of his environment. But here, in addition, there is often a period of confusion after the child stops staring. Also, during the spell, he may get up and wander around the room, pick at his clothes, and fail to respond appropriately. These "peculiar" episodes are likely to be misunderstood by the other children in the classroom and by his teacher. As with absence spells, it is important that the teacher understands what is happening. The teacher needs to realize that if your child is wandering around and someone tries to restrain him, the child may lash out or even become highly agitated. Providing gentle guidance and supervision at such times is far better than trying to make him sit down. The teacher needs to be able to be comforting and reassuring both to the student, who is not aware of what is happening, and to the other children, who may be confused by the behavior. It is important that the teacher alert you to changes in your child's performance. You can then alert your doctor.

As with other recurrent seizures, your child needs to understand what is happening during these episodes when he is not aware. He may remember the beginning of the seizure, when he felt the aura (for example, fear, rising feeling in the stomach), and he may be vaguely aware of people responding to his behavior during and after the seizure. Or he may only be aware that something happened and that now things are different from what they were a few seconds or minutes ago. Since these spells usually follow a pattern, let him know what has been going on so that he will be less upset and confused. If he does have an aura, point out that it can be a useful warning. Encourage him to pay attention so that he can avoid harmful situations.

## Is Your Child Disabled or Handicapped?

No, there is life with and after epilepsy. Let's talk about the important things in your child's life—about all the times when he is *not* having seizures.

Society glibly says that everybody should be able to do what he wants if he tries hard enough. Clearly this is foolishness! Some people are too short to be basketball players. Others are too tall to be jockeys. Some people are not beautiful enough to be movie stars. Some wear glasses and can't, therefore, be astronauts. In this global sense all of us are handicapped. However, we should all have the opportunity to achieve our full potential, whatever that may be. Neither society, nor parents, nor our own attitudes should be allowed to interfere with this.

Is epilepsy a "handicap"? For some it clearly is. For most, it need not be. The child whose seizures are now well controlled with medicine need not be handicapped. He can achieve his full potential, even if there will be some limitations in his choices. Crucial for your child's future is that you not impose unreasonable limitations on his activities or aspirations, nor allow others to do so.

### "Can I let my child go out and play?"

Of course! You not only can, but must let him go out and play, go on trips, sleep at a friend's house. "But suppose he has another seizure?" That's a risk you have to take. A careful analysis of risks is an important part of raising any child. It is a particularly important part of raising a child with the uncertainties of epilepsy. It is the crucial ingredient in avoiding overprotection. His ability to run around and his intelligence are the same as before the seizures. Most children with epilepsy are neither retarded or learning-disabled. For most such children, the only impairment is that, from time to time, there may be a seizure. For 99.99 percent of the time your child is the same as always.

"BUT ISN'T HE DISABLED?" The answer is NO! He can still run and play, go to school, sleep over at a friend's house. There is virtually *nothing* that a child who has had a few seizures cannot do. "Can he ride a bike?" Sure. The chances of having a seizure while riding his bike are very small; he is only minimally at greater risk than before his seizures. "Can she swim?" Absolutely, but her swimming must be supervised, just as every child's swimming must be supervised. "Isn't there a higher risk that she could drown or have a seizure in the water?" Yes, but only a *slightly* higher risk, since she has had only occasional seizures and may never have another one. Technically, your child may have a disability. He or she may fit the government definition that enables a person to obtain special services if the seizures interfere with education or work. But having a disability is very different from being disabled.

A handicap is often superimposed by society, parents, friends, or schools. A person can also impose it on himself.

We find that the best approach to a child who has had several seizures, who has now been labeled "epileptic," is for you to gain a realistic acceptance of your child's limitations (if any) and to focus on his potential. This requires a conscious effort to put aside your anxiety and concern about all of the things that could happen. This is not an easy thing to do. It requires acceptance of the fact that there are risks inherent in rearing any child and that most children with epilepsy, especially those whose epilepsy is controlled, face only slightly greater risks than other children.

Children who have severe, or intractable, epilepsy and those who have additional impairments such as mental retardation, cerebral palsy, or learning disabilities also require realistic acceptance. It is equally important that these children, too, be encouraged to reach their full potential, and that additional handicaps not be superimposed (see Chapter 16).

# 15. Coping with the Uncertainties of Seizures and Epilepsy:
## The Power of Positive Thinking

## A Tale of Two Parents

❑ Melanie's mother was thirty-two and had struggled hard to achieve this, her first pregnancy. She was, naturally, quite anxious when she went into premature labor and delivered a three-pound baby girl. Problems with breathing led to Melanie's immediate transfer to University Hospital. Dr. Richards, Melanie's intern, seemed very competent and conscientious. After a thorough examination, and after Melanie was settled in the isolette with all the tubes and the respirator, the doctor spent a lot of time with Melanie's father explaining the problems and the potential problems of a premature infant. She told him that it was really too early to predict the outcome, and that most children with such respiratory problems could be saved without permanent lung disease. Other problems could occur: intestinal problems, seizures, bleeding into the head. "Small babies like this can have a greater chance of mental retardation, cerebral palsy, and epilepsy," she said. "However," she reassured him, "at the moment Melanie looks very good. We have reason to be hopeful."

Mr. White relayed this information to his wife. The nurses at the community hospital tried to be as reassuring as possible. They all had seen premature infants who had done well. On the fourth day, Mrs. White was discharged and was able to see her daughter for the first time. Melanie was unbelievably tiny, but Dr. Richards again reassured her that everything was going well, so far. Actually, the next five weeks in the hospital nursery went very well. Melanie did not develop any major complications. She grew and thrived and went home weighing four-and-one-half pounds.

This should have been the end of a happy story, but it is the beginning of another tale—or rather two different tales: one is the mother's, the other the father's.

Mrs. White was an accountant for a prominent firm in town and had worked very hard to achieve her senior position. Indeed, this was one of the reasons she had deferred having children. She was also a worrier. The doctor had mentioned the possibility of mental retardation and cerebral palsy. "Is Melanie all right?" she would repeatedly ask her pediatrician. "Shouldn't she be smiling by now?" "When should she be rolling over?" Reassurance that premature babies were a bit slower to do these things only made Mrs. White more anxious, particularly when she saw other infants beginning to sit at six months and walk around furniture before they were a year old.

Melanie was able to sit when she was ten months old, began cruising around furniture when she was fourteen months, and said her first words at about a year. "All of these are normal, particularly for a baby who was born five weeks prematurely," the pediatrician said. But Mrs. White knew that they were at the lower end of normal and she worried. "Isn't she supposed to be using her thumb and index finger to be feeding herself by now?" she would ask. "I think that her right foot turns out when she walks. Is that normal? I'd like to take Melanie to the pediatric orthopedist to see if she has CP."

Mr. White was a college professor who did much of his writing and research at home. By nature, he was more laid back and less of a worrier. He spent a lot of time with Melanie while his wife was at work, and he thought that Melanie was just fine. "Einstein did not talk until he was three," he was fond of reminding his wife.

The orthopedist found no deformities. "She's just a little slow in gaining control of her muscles," he said. "She'll be walking soon," and she did.

When, at two, Melanie had a cold and a sore throat, she experienced a convulsion. It was over before the ambulance got there, and the pediatrician met them at the hospital's emergency room. After an examination, he reassured them that this was a febrile seizure and that she would be fine. He said she did not need medication because there was only one chance in about three of her having another febrile seizure. Mr. White was delighted that Melanie did not need medication. By contrast, his wife thought that one in three was a lot and was less happy, particularly when her daughter had a second convulsion with fever four months later. An EEG, done to assuage Mrs. White's concern, was normal, but Melanie was placed on phenobarbital "to prevent still another one." Unfortunately, phenobarbital made Melanie a terror. She was irritable, overactive, fussy, and had problems going to sleep. After two weeks, everyone agreed that she was far better without the medicine, and it was stopped.

When she entered nursery school at three, Melanie seemed less mature than her peers. She was less ready to play in the groups, less interested in hearing stories, not as good at coloring within the lines. The teachers expressed their concerns at the parents' conference. Mr. White's reaction was: "Let's keep her in the play group another year. There's no need for her to be the youngest in the next group. In another year she'll be older, wiser, and more mature. After all, she did start this world early." Mrs. White insisted on psychological testing; it showed that Melanie was "low normal," more like a two-and-one-half-year-old than her chronological age of three years and four months. The report also stated that "Melanie's strengths are in the personal-social area. In fine motor coordination and the perceptual areas she lags slightly behind." A visit to the pediatric neurologist confirmed that she was not mentally retarded and that she did not have cerebral palsy. "She is just slightly slow in development, as are many premature babies. They usually catch up as they enter school."

Melanie's mother found a speech therapist who would see the child at about five in the afternoon, so that she herself wouldn't have to leave work early. She and her husband would alternate taking Melanie for therapy and practicing speech sounds. An occupational therapist also saw her once a week, and Mrs. White found a Saturday morning gym class for "exceptional children." She considered that "together time."

When they first came to our office, Melanie was five and had just had her first generalized, non-febrile seizure. Most of the questions came from her mother. "Why did she have a seizure? Will she have another? Shouldn't she be on medication? Can she still go to the gym class? They do all these exercises swinging on bars. What about riding her bike?" They were the questions you may have asked your own physician. Mr. White had few questions; he mainly listened as we tried to explain seizures and the uncertainties of the future.

"Why can't you doctors ever give a straight answer to a simple question?" Mrs. White finally cried out in anguish. "I thought you were supposed to be scientific." We tried again. We explained the potential side effects of treatment, and they agreed not to start treatment at this time. Every week or so, Mrs. White would call our coordinator to describe one thing or another. "Melanie was sucking her thumb, and I had to call her three times before she responded. Is that the absence seizures the doctor mentioned might occur?" "Melanie has fallen twice this week and skinned her knee. How do you tell if she just tripped or if this was an akinetic seizure?" "The teacher tells me that Melanie is not paying attention in school this week. Could she be having seizures, or do you think it is just her cold?" "I was watching while she was sleeping last night and she was really very restless. Could these be seizures during her sleep?"

"This is driving my wife crazy," Mr. White told us on one visit. "I think that Melanie is doing fine. She's a delicate flower who is just taking her own time to bloom. She is sweet, lovable, affectionate, but my wife is so concerned about seizures, and about Melanie's future, that she's unable to enjoy her any more. She's stopped worrying about the mental retardation and cerebral palsy, or at least she's not focusing on those things any more, but the uncertainty about future seizures and about what is or is not a seizure is affecting my wife's work. It's ruining our marriage, and it's hurting Melanie. We've got a wonderful little girl here, and my wife is spending so much time being concerned that she's missing all the fun."

When Melanie had a second generalized seizure one year later, things got even worse. She was started on medication, and concerns about the side ef- fects were added to the confusion about what were and what were not seizures and the fears about the possibility of injury when she was out playing. The already troubled marriage was now more so. Melanie herself became more manipulative. When she did not get her way, she would sulk and stare. Was she having an absence seizure? With her mother's fear of the effects of punishment, of getting Mellanie upset and causing another seizure, Melanie's behavior grew worse. Problems she experienced in learning to read in the first grade led to concerns about the possible effect of the medication on her learning ability, and then to changes in medication. During the change-over, Melanie had a complex partial seizure, and this, in turn, led to additional concerns.

The frequent visits to our clinic became increasingly difficult for everyone. We couldn't satisfy Mrs. White, because we could not give categorical answers to her questions. "Was this the best medicine?" We could only answer that this medicine worked on many children with this type of seizure and did not often have serious side effects. "But how do you know that Melanie wouldn't do better on _____?" "We don't, but this is what we would choose first." We would try to point out the potential risks and benefits of switching. "Will she have another tonic-clonic seizure?" We would reexplain the uncertainties of epilep- sy. "If we take her to visit my parents in Alabama, what do we do if she has a seizure during the long drive?" "Could she die during a seizure if she had one during the night?" "How do we know that she isn't having seizures during the night that we are not aware of?" The questions were endless, as were the doubts, and both were unanswerable.

Two or three years of counseling, and of patiently answering and reanswering the same questions, and also of marriage counseling finally led to acceptance of the facts. Melanie was a lovely young lady—beautiful, well-dressed, very sociable. She was an adequate student who required special resource teaching, a little slow, the lower end of normal, but not retarded. She was not graceful, but participated in a children's ballet class. We would have called her a child with learning disabilities and sort of "clumsy," with what neurologists call "soft neurological signs." We would not have dignified her minimal deficits by calling them either cerebral palsy or mental retardation. Melanie's seizures remained under control with medication.

Mrs. White finally came to accept the state of affairs and to accept Melanie for what she is, not for what she once hoped she would be. And what she was, on her own terms, was terrific. How much easier those years were for Mr. White, who had accepted her on those terms all along.

In all chronic conditions there is a need to "be realistic" and a problem in defining "reality" and in accepting it. One of the most difficult realities of epilepsy is that no one can predict when and where (or even if) a next seizure will occur. This is "the uncertainty factor." It is this uncertainty factor that differentiates epilepsy from most other chronic conditions. It is this uncertainty factor that is most disturbing to older children with epilepsy as well as to their parents. "Could I have a seizure while crossing the street?" "Is it all right for me to go to school today, or will I be embarrassed by another one of those things?" "Suppose he goes to the prom and has a seizure?" Uncertainty leads to anxiety and worry. Coping with anxiety is the principal task for a parent of a child with epilepsy. Worry must be contained. It cannot be allowed to permeate every waking moment of your life. It cannot be allowed to be the master, dictating overprotection of your child.

But how can worry and anxiety be contained? It's useless to be told not to worry. You need to be helped to see the reality of your child's epilepsy. For some, that reality may be a few seizures, likely to be controlled, and epilepsy that eventually disappears. For other parents, the reality may be continuing seizures or retardation or other disabilities. No one can predict with absolute certainty what the future holds for a child with epilepsy, any more than we can predict with certainty what the future holds for a child without epilepsy.

It is the lack of ability to influence the future that can be the most disturbing to people with epilepsy and to their loved ones.

## The Power of Positive Thinking

One way to achieve a positive approach to dealing with this uncertainty is to focus on the low probability of another seizure. A second way is to recognize that another seizure may occur and accept that possibility. It's important to find what approach works for you and your child to lead you to acceptance.

You might say to yourself: "She's going to be one of the lucky ones with benign epilepsy who will, or has, outgrown it." Or you might say, "Chances are that she will *never* have another seizure." Never is a long time and it might be more useful to say, "She's not going to have another seizure today." If you said that to yourself, the chances are overwhelming that you would be correct. If you said, "I don't think she will have another seizure this week or this month," you still have an enormous chance of being right. Many people with epilepsy have only two, or three, or four seizures in their lifetimes.

If you live your life *as if* your child is not going to have another seizure, then you can avoid the extra handicap superimposed by worrying about another seizure and its possible effects. If you allow your child to live as if another seizure will never occur, you can avoid the overprotection that may accompany the fear that it will. Thinking that another seizure will not occur can be called "denial." But it is not denial that your child has epilepsy. For many people, at most times, denial that another seizure will occur will be realistic. Most of the time you will have been correct.

What happens if your confidence is wrong and your child has another seizure? You and your physician will explore why that seizure occurred. Did your child forget her medicine? Not enough sleep? Does she have an infection? Does the medication need adjusting? You may find a good reason. If you don't, you will have to begin your power of positive thinking all over again.

However, you'll be right about her not having a seizure far more often than you'll be wrong. And, since the consequences of being wrong are not within your control, this framework may help you and your child achieve a positive approach to living.

Another approach involves the realization that medical risks of a recurrent seizure are minimal and that, as in the past, your child will quickly recover from the seizure to resume his normal activities. You may even be able to accept the social consequences and not be overly concerned that you or your child will experience embarrassment. It may be easier for your child to do this if she has a good understanding of seizures and if you have been able to educate her school and her friends that although having a seizure is unpleasant and interrupts activities for a short while, these activities usually can be resumed without any real harm.

Different people use different methods of coping, and some may need to use more than one. Your physicians and other advisors may recommend that you try a particular approach, but you and your child will have to find your own way to minimize anxiety and to cope. ANXIETY IS PERHAPS THE GREATEST ENEMY OF PEOPLE WITH SEIZURES.

## Anxiety, the Greatest Enemy

Coping with anxiety is a crucial step in acceptance of your child and her problem. You may have sensed the teacher's anxiety when you first told her about your child's seizures, or perhaps you simply worried how she might react. Maybe her anxiety is a consequence of lack of information. Perhaps she has been exposed to the myths. Perhaps she once had a child in her classroom who fell and hit his head during a seizure. You may be able to reassure the teacher by saying, "I know that you're worried that Steve will fall and be injured and that I'll be furious and accuse you of not looking out for him. But I won't. We'll both be upset that it happened. But we both have to realize that Steve needs to be in school with his classmates. His seizures are really infrequent, and he usually has a little warning. We need to convince him to let you know that warning has come so that he can be in a safe place. We have to let him take some chances if he's to have the opportunity to be a normal child."

This kind of dialogue is critical to an understanding and working relationship between parent, child, and teacher. Teachers often need help in coming to terms with their anxiety, just as you do. Acceptance of the realities and accurate information can do a lot to relieve anxiety for everyone. When you have come to believe what you just said, you have come a long way in accepting your child and his epilepsy.

There is a common saying that admonishes us to accept with serenity the things that cannot be changed, to have the courage to change the things that can be changed, and to have the wisdom to know the difference. If your child's seizures have been controlled, acceptance of the reality that your child is back to his normal state is easier. If your child continues to have seizures, you may not be able to change that reality. If so, you and your child must have the courage to change your own perception of that reality and to help change the perceptions of others.

One kind of acceptance, however, is totally unacceptable. It is virtually never appropriate to accept that your child must be significantly limited by his seizures. You have to believe that your child can fulfill his own potential. If learning problems or physical problems exist, they must be recognized and solutions sought to optimize your child's ability to function.

Realistic acceptance of the multiple handicapped child is crucial. This does not mean that this acceptance should not incorporate a positive attitude, or that hope should be lost. Seizures that were intractable only a few years ago may respond to new medications, or to new combinations of medications, or to surgery today or tomorrow. Focusing on what your child can do now rather than on what he cannot do, looking at the glass as half-full, rather than half-empty, will help you and your child through the rough times. Encouraging the child to be able to say, "I'm all right now, I can go back to class" or "I know that I had a seizure, but now I want to go out to play" are all part of the same positive outlook. A positive attitude discourages the invalidism that can accompany a chronic disability. It encourages your child to have as much control as possible over his life. It maximizes his self-esteem.

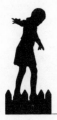

# 16. Coping with Substantial Handicap:
# Mental Retardation, Cerebral Palsy, Intractable Seizures

For 80 percent of children with epilepsy, seizures can be controlled. For those children and their families, epilepsy is not and should not be a substantial handicap. For 20 percent, the uncontrolled seizures themselves may constitute a significant impairment; and for some children with mental retardation or cerebral palsy, epilepsy may be a substantial secondary disability. These children and their parents carry a significant burden, a greater degree of guilt, anger, frustration, sorrow, and just plain hard work. These parents need to understand these disabilities so they may help their children as much as circumstances allow.

Damage to the brain causes these problems. Damage in the motor areas of the brain causes cerebral palsy. When damage or dysfunction occurs throughout a considerable area of the brain it may lead to mental retardation. Epilepsy also exists because the brain is not functioning properly. Mental retardation and cerebral palsy, while sometimes accompanied by epilepsy, never cause epilepsy. Epilepsy never causes cerebral palsy and seldom causes mental retardation.

Parents with a severely disabled child must also gradually come to a realistic acceptance of their child's disability. Mechanisms for coping are the same as for the parent of the less disabled child, but the goal is often far more difficult to achieve. In addition to working through your own adjustment, you must also help your child get the service he will

**Table 16.1 Terminology, IQ, and Academic and Vocational Potential of Children with Mental Retardation**

| Degree of mental retardation | IQ (approximate) | Academic potential* | Vocational potential |
|---|---|---|---|
| None | >80 | Normal | Normal |
| Borderline | 70–79 | 6th grade level | Employable |
| Mild | 55–70 | 4th grade level | Employable |
| Moderate | 40–55 | May read and write simple words | Non-competitive employment |
| Severe | 25–40 | | Sheltered/supported "employment" |
| Profound | <25 | | |

*Modified from* H. J. Cohen, "Mental Retardation." In H. M. Wallace, R. F. Biehl, *et al.,* eds. *Handicapped Children and Youth.* (New York: Human Sciences Press: 1987), p. 354.
    *Academic potential levels cited are approximations; function will vary within each group and with each individual child.

need. You must be an advocate. Both you and your child will have special needs. Finding the help is sometimes difficult; for some people, accepting the help is even more difficult.

## Mental Retardation

By definition, mental retardation is a handicapping condition defined as less than average intelligence, less than average personal independence and social responsibility. Ninety-seven out of 100 children have an intelligence score of 70–130; children with mental retardation have scores that are less than 70. (See Table 16.1 for the terminology used for the levels of retardation, IQ, and the approximate expected academic and vocational function at each level.)

In a child who is already handicapped by retardation, seizures can further impair function and require treatment. Except in the severely brain-damaged child, seizures are as readily controlled as in a child of normal intelligence.

Parents of children with substantial handicaps necessarily are deeply concerned. They are perplexed by many questions, among them the following:

*"If my child is mentally retarded, what are her chances
of developing epilepsy?"*

About one in ten children with mental retardation also have epilepsy. The figure itself is, however, virtually meaningless since the risk of epilepsy varies markedly with the cause of retardation, its severity, and the age of the child. The severely or profoundly retarded child is far more likely to have seizures than the mildly retarded child. With children who are severely retarded, seizures are likely to begin, if they begin at all, in infancy or early childhood.

The child whose retardation is caused by brain trauma or lack of oxygen, sustained either during birth or later, is more likely to have seizures than a child whose retardation has an unknown cause. Severe retardation of genetic origin has a significantly different risk of epilepsy depending on the specific cause. In one condition, Rett's syndrome, epilepsy occurs almost universally; in Down's syndrome, however, the risk of seizures is only slightly higher than average.

*"If my child has epilepsy, what is the chance of mental retardation?"*

The risk of retardation in a child with epilepsy depends primarily on the cause of the epilepsy and to a far less extent on the type of seizure itself. A previously normal child who begins to have seizures of unknown cause will virtually never become retarded. However, if these seizures are caused by a progressive or degenerative disease, the risk of retardation is higher. Children with developmental delay or neurological handicap seldom become more retarded because of seizures, the two exceptions being infants with infantile spasms and children with the Lennox-Gastaut syndrome. Both of these types of epilepsy are usually associated with progressive retardation.

## Coping with Labels

Everybody gets labelled. Some are labelled beautiful. Some are labelled dumb. These labels are undefined and, therefore, basically useless. If your child were labelled artistic, however, and as a result got into special art classes, that label would have been useful. A label of normal is not useful if a child's learning style makes it difficult to learn in a normal class. He is denied the special help he needs. A label of mild or moderate mental retardation will be useful if the child is placed in a classroom that meets his special needs. But to put him in a class with other moderately retarded children does not alone meet his needs. All moderate retardation is not the same, just as all epilepsy is not. Labels can miscategorize and stigmatize a child. Will a label be an advantage to your child? If a label of "green" helps your child get the appropriate services, it will be a useful label.

It is important that your expectations for your child are realistic. Putting a handicapped child in a regular class may or may not be to his advantage. Mainstreaming has many advantages, but it may be a disadvantage for an individual child. The stress may be overwhelming.

*The most important thing for your child is to get the appropriate services that he needs so that he can fulfill his own potential.*

**"I don't believe my child is retarded; I think his problems are due to all those medicines he's taking. How can I tell for sure?"**

Parents may prefer to believe that a child's slowness is a result of the medication, but the effects of medication overdose seldom resemble mental retardation. Children with retardation tend to progress at their own rate, while drug toxicity usually causes a decline in function. Over-medicated children often are sleepy during the day or unsteady; mentally retarded children are neither.

The only way to rule out dosage as a cause is to decrease or eliminate one or all of the drugs in use. Do not do this on your own. With your physician's advice, you may want to consider tapering medication slowly, decreasing a single type of medication at a time. *If*, on tapering medicine, your child's function obviously improves, *then* the slowing, or a portion of the retardation, *may* have been drug related. You and your physician will have to decide whether the risk of decreasing or changing the medication, as well as the chance of recurring or worsening seizures, is outweighed by the possible benefit of improved intellectual function.

Barbiturates like phenobarbital and benzodiazepines like diazepam (Valium), clonazepam (Klonopin), clorazepate (Tranxene), or lorazepam (Ativan) may cause slowness, dullness, sleepiness, and depression, symptoms that may resemble the characteristics of retardation. Any anticonvulsant, even when in the therapeutic range, may, on occasion, interfere with mental function.

**"How should I treat my child who has both retardation and epilepsy?"**

The answer depends on the child's level of retardation. The natural tendency of most parents and grandparents is to overprotect a child

with epilepsy. However, overprotection, particularly of a mentally retarded child, leads to infantilization, ultimately a greater handicap to a
child than the seizures themselves. It is crucial for such a child to be as
independent as possible. The retarded child needs every opportunity to
achieve his optimal potential.

When your child has multiple problems, such as mental retardation
and epilepsy, the family has a lot of compensating to do. With epilepsy
alone, you can usually maintain your expectations for his future—
assuming, of course, they were realistic to begin with—since most
epilepsy can be controlled or outgrown. Even when epilepsy occurs in
children with retardation, your expectations for your child should
rarely be changed.

Helping your child to cope with mental retardation depends greatly
on the degree of retardation. The severely retarded child may not be
clearly aware of his disability. Today many moderately retarded individuals function in noncompetitive employment, are able to live in the
community with assistance, and engage in a variety of social activities.
The process of developing these capabilities begins in childhood with
mainstreaming in schools and socialization through churches, scout-
ing, and athletics. Developing these capabilities begins within the family as well—seeing a child's potential, encouraging him to learn to
participate, helping him to achieve his full worth.

## Cerebral Palsy

Cerebral palsy (CP) is a condition in which the body's control of
motor movements or posture is abnormal. It is caused by damage
within the motor areas of the brain or spinal cord that has occurred
before or during birth or during childhood. It is not caused by a tumor
or by degeneration of the nervous system. Cerebral palsy is not progressive; it does not continue to become worse, although it may become
more obvious or its symptoms may vary slightly as the child matures.

### "Will my child who has cerebral palsy be retarded? Will he have epilepsy?"

Not quite half of the children with cerebral palsy are retarded to
some degree; a number of others may have behavior and learning problems. A number have no such problems, and are of normal intelligence;
indeed, some have superior intelligence.

Table 16.2 Types of Cerebral Palsy and Risks of Seizures

| Type | Frequency (approximate % of all cases) | Risk of seizures |
|---|---|---|
| Stiff (spastic) | | |
| Both legs (diplegia) | 30.0 | Low |
| One-sided (hemiparesis) | 25.0 | Moderate |
| Both sides (quadriparesis) | 25.0 | High |
| Abnormal movements (dyskinesia) | 10.0 | Low |
| Athetoid | N.A. | N.A. |
| Dystonic | N.A. | N.A. |
| Mixed (spastic and dyskinesia) | 10.0 | Variable |

Approximately one in three children with cerebral palsy will also have epilepsy, but few children with epilepsy will have cerebral palsy. *Epilepsy does not cause cerebral palsy; it does not cause mental retardation. Nor does cerebral palsy cause epilepsy. When cerebral palsy and epilepsy do occur together, underlying damage to the brain has caused both.*

There are various forms of cerebral palsy, and the present classification is far from satisfactory. (One scheme for classification is shown in Table 16.2.) It indicates, broadly, that both the frequency and type of seizures vary with the kind of cerebral palsy, as discussed below.

## Spastic Hemiparesis

A spastic hemiparesis is a form of cerebral palsy that affects only one side of the body. It is caused by damage in the opposite side of the brain by a stroke, bleeding into the brain, trauma, or a problem in the brain's development. The arm is usually more affected than the leg; there may be major problems with the use of the hand. Such children will usually be able to learn to walk with a limp. Since the damage is focal (one-sided), these individuals are less likely to have mental retardation. Although we do not understand all of the factors that cause one person's damaged brain to provoke seizures while another's does not, and cannot predict which child will have seizures and which will not, in general we do know that a child with a hemiparesis whose CT or MRI scan shows brain damage is more likely to have seizures than one who does not have these problems. We treat the seizures as we do other focal seizures. Unlike the child with a spastic quadraparesis, the child with a hemiparesis may be a candidate for focal epilepsy surgery to remove the damaged tissue causing the seizures if they are uncontrollable.

## Spastic Quadriparesis

Children with stiffness in all four limbs (spastic quadraparesis) usually have sustained severe damage to the entire brain. They are likely to have severe or even profound retardation. They often have experienced seizures in the newborn period (see neonatal seizures) and may have had infantile spasms during the first year of life. They will have a high incidence of generalized tonic-clonic seizures as well as of atonic attacks and the Lennox-Gastaut syndrome. Seizures in children with spastic quadraparesis may be very difficult to control.

## Diplegia

Diplegia is the type of cerebral palsy in which both legs are stiff. It is far more common in children who were born prematurely than children carried to full term. These children are usually of normal intelligence and are less likely to develop seizures. Their principal handicap is a difficulty with walking; physical therapy, bracing, and orthopedic surgery can often be of help.

## Abnormal Movements

When brain damage affects areas of the brain that control the coordination of movements, the child may be athetoid; movements are performed slowly and in a writhing fashion. Damage to other areas of the brain may cause more rigid movements, that is, dystonia. Since these control areas lie deep within the brain in regions less likely to cause seizures, epilepsy is uncommon among such children. They are also less likely to be retarded.

Children with damage to multiple areas of the brain may have both spasticity and either athetosis or dystonia. Such children are said to have mixed cerebral palsy.

### *"How can I help my child who has cerebral palsy?"*

Helping your child to cope with cerebral palsy depends on whether or not there is mental retardation. Many children with cerebral palsy are of normal intelligence, and for these children the motor dysfunction can be enormously frustrating. To be unable to dress, to go to the bathroom alone, to feed yourself can create such a sense of helplessness and dependence that depression is not uncommon. And yet children with cerebral palsy are increasingly able to find areas in which they can become competent and ultimately develop self-esteem. Appropriate use of computers allows both learning and communication. Motorized wheelchairs and special adaptations may permit mobility and independence. It is amazing what can be done to help unlock the real person who is within.

For the child with cerebral palsy as for the child with mental retardation the most important ingredients in successfully coping are development of motivation and self-esteem. Motivation can be stimulated by activities and hard work such as those involved in preparing for the Special Olympics. The joy of successfully participating in such sports promotes self-esteem. Special Olympics is a model of what can be achieved in other areas of life, with patience and persistence. Such children need role models of successful handicapped adults. Their ability to become an achieving adult begins with small successes in the family and in the school.

Helping your handicapped child to cope with the accompanying psychological problems is still an art, not a science. How to do this is unclear, but he, and you also, need help in articulating your frustrations, concerns, your anger, and your hopes.

There has been amazing progress in recent years in enabling both the retarded and those with cerebral palsy to participate more fully in the community. The old stereotypes of institutionalization and handicap persist. But these children, while *dis*-abled, are not *un*-able.

## Intractable Seizures

For most children seizures are not uncontrollable, they are only intractable, that is, difficult to control. There is good reason to hope for control. The next medicine may be successful or a combination of medications may bring control. Surgery may offer a solution. You may need to get a second opinion, and you may decide to consult with an epilepsy specialist or an epilepsy center. Many times parents of children with intractable seizures who persisted in looking for the right therapy have turned uncontrollable seizures into controlled seizures.

❑ Margo was a bright ten-year-old with intractable seizures. Her hemiparesis was not disabling, but several seizures each week and the effects of all of her medications were interfering with her progress. She came to us looking for surgery to remove the epileptic focus. Unfortunately, we found that there were abnormal areas on both sides of the brain and surgery was not an option. She had had good trials of virtually all of the anticonvulsants. After a lot of discussion with her parents and with her, and despite her age, we decided to try the ketogenic diet. Margo said she would do almost anything to get rid of those darn seizures. It's been over a year now. Margo has faithfully stuck to the diet. She has had no seizures. She is off all of her medications and is doing superbly well.

Families need to persist in looking for a solution, and physicians also need to be willing to keep trying. Both need to be willing to take risks to achieve benefits. Unfortunately, not every family finds such a happy ending.

❑ Greg is a fifteen-year-old boy whose seizures began in early childhood. Although his development was delayed, seizures came under control with medication and the family was able to adjust to their mildly retarded son. At age five, the seizures recurred and Greg appeared more severely delayed. The family again went through grieving, anger, and frustration while the physicians tried new medications. Eventually the seizures were again controlled and the family readjusted to their new circumstances. At age nine, atonic seizures began and Greg made frequent trips to the emergency room for stitches. During the brief periods of time when these seizures were brought under control, Greg could function in the moderately retarded range. But the frequency of seizures or the side effects of medication continued to handicap him. An abnormality on the MRI scan led us to hope that surgery might control his seizures. Surgery was successful even though his minimal hemiparesis increased. Greg only had rare seizures in his sleep. He wasn't falling, and his language and function had improved. Both his family and Greg were delighted. This honeymoon lasted for six months until the seizures recurred.

In Greg's case we and the family have a dilemma. We know of no other combination of medicines likely to control his seizures. We are considering further surgery to section the corpus callosum. Will further surgery be of benefit? Are the risks of new surgery worth taking? What are the chances of success? The answers are unclear.

There are many lessons in Greg's story. One lesson is that even if parents do develop a realistic acceptance of their child's limitations, that acceptance may be challenged when the situation changes. Adjustment for those families whose children have multiple handicaps may be a roller coaster. A second lesson is that often other approaches might succeed in controlling intractable seizures. Deciding whether or not to take the risks of these new approaches when you don't know their benefits in advance can be difficult for both the family and the concerned physician. There may be a time when you and your physician must accept the status quo, but the question will be, when has that time come?

## Coping with Severe Handicap with Epilepsy

A parent may come to accept the limitations, even the severe limitations, of cerebral palsy or mental retardation, realizing that there is no medicine or surgery that can reverse cerebral palsy or mental retardation. "But if you could only get rid of the seizures," you may say to us, "life would not be so difficult. I thought you could control seizures with medicine for most children. Why is my child still having seizures?"

Seizures in a child who has other evidence of brain damage may be much more difficult to control. Still, your physician should try new medications, and even if your child is retarded, surgery may not be impossible. You may need to find a physician who is willing to consider new options.

If your child's damage is primarily in one portion of the brain, removal of that portion could be of benefit. However, most children who are retarded have damage on both sides of the brain; removal of one portion will not be of benefit. Still, even in the child who has bilateral brain damage, section of the corpus callosum can sometimes be of benefit in controlling the atonic seizures that lead to injury, although this surgery, in the severely brain-injured child, has a lower rate of success.

Why do we treat seizures? We treat seizures because they interfere with a child's function. For the otherwise normal child, occasional seizures that interfere with function require treatment. For the severely handicapped child, however, an occasional seizure may be less handicapping than the toxicity of medications. The risks of treatment and its potential benefits must, therefore, be evaluated carefully in light of your

child's other handicaps. When seizures interfere with your child's behavior or interfere with placement in otherwise optimal programs in
school, every effort reasonable should be made to control them. Schools
may be reluctant to accept the responsibility of a child who has seizures.
Parents should first try to convince the school that the seizures are not a
major problem. It will require persistence, information, and lobbying.
If necessary, it may take legal action. The solution will require both
strong advocacy and compromise.

❏ Katie was two-and-a-half and severely handicapped. She functioned like
a one-year-old. She was not able to walk or talk. Fortunately, her local school
system had a superb program for handicapped children. This program had
occupational therapists, physical therapists, and speech therapists. Katie was
an ideal candidate—except for her seizures. The school claimed that they had
no one who could cope with her frequent generalized tonic-clonic seizures.
What would happen if a seizure was prolonged? What were they to do? Katie
would require far more time than the other children, and if a seizure occurred,
they had no one with the special training needed. Katie's mother had no problem coping with her child's seizures, although she had had no special training.
To put it frankly, the school was afraid of accepting the responsibility. Katie was
deprived of her right to an optimal program. The school's solution was a home
teaching program with visits several times a week. Clearly this was not optimal.
Finally we helped Katie's mother to achieve a compromise. She agreed to go to
school to handle the seizures while the teachers taught. Over several weeks the
school came to realize that Katie's seizures did not pose a major problem, and
no longer required that her mother be present.

The end of Katie's story was that she was found to be a candidate for
surgery, her damaged hemisphere was removed, and she no longer has
seizures.

## A Parent's Special Needs

As parent of a child with severe disability you have special needs as
well. We have talked about success stories, the child who has been cured
of his seizures. Magazines are full of such success stories. The epilepsy
movement has concentrated on a message of hope in its campaign to
eliminate the stigma associated with epilepsy. But for parents of multiply handicapped children, or children with intractable seizures, the

message of hope is frustrating. These parents feel left out of the main-stream. They are angry, worried that their children will not get the help they need, and fearful that they themselves will be unable to cope.

### *"My God! How do I cope with all this?"*

You need help! Every parent needs help in a situation like this. Each faces a terrible feeling of loneliness when confronted with the over-whelming dual problems, for example, of mental retardation and epi-lepsy. The initial stages of grieving, denial, and anger that any parent with a disabled child experiences are compounded by a feeling of shame, of wanting to tell no one, of feeling that you are the only person in the world who has faced such overwhelming problems. Nor do you want to bother your physician with your sense of hopelessness. "He is always too busy." Or maybe the way he has explained things to you has simply confused you. "Did he really say . . . ?"

There are several places to turn. *First,* give your doctor another chance. Ask him to explain again. *Write down your questions* before you ask them because, in the stress and intimidation of an office visit, anyone can forget what questions they wanted to ask. A second place to turn is the local affiliate of the Epilepsy Foundation of America. There are many such affiliates around the country. If you have difficulty finding one, contact the national office of the Epilepsy Foundation of America (EFA) in Landover, Maryland. Their toll-free number is 1–800–EFA–1000; in Maryland call 301–539–3700. Either the local chapter or the national office can provide information that will answer your questions.

A third and important step is to contact a local support group. Since your child has mental retardation or cerebral palsy as well as epilepsy, a local organization for retarded citizens or for individuals with cerebral palsy can be immensely helpful.

### *"I don't want to be part of a group. I don't need them, and I don't need to hear about someone else's problems. I have enough of my own."*

We often hear this statement from parents. Or else one parent will say, "I'd like to go, but my husband (wife) won't have anything to do with it." Groups are generally helpful, but some people are just not ready to join a group at a particular time in their lives. Some people are embarrassed to talk about their feelings or problems in public. But you are not the only one who has had to deal with such problems. Hearing how other parents have coped is often far more helpful than hearing similar advice from your physician. Parents choose different words, have a different tone to what they say. And they have "lived" it, not just learned about it. Talking about your problems can help put them in perspective.

If you feel you do not need a group, or feel that you can't cope with counseling just now, reconsider it later. Remember: If you have adjusted so well that you can't use any help, perhaps you have a responsibility to join a group so that you can help someone else.

Children who have both cerebral palsy and/or mental retardation as well as epilepsy need considerable support. And so do their families. The combination of these disabilities may seem overwhelming, but remember you are not alone. There are many organizations to help you and available services. Every child, regardless of disability, is entitled to an appropriate education, for example. Handicapped children are eligible to receive services as soon as their handicaps have been identified, at whatever age. Ask your doctor, your school system, or your local health department about these services. You don't have to wait until your child is old enough for school.

For the child who has cerebral palsy, and for the parent of that child, United Cerebral Palsy (UCP) provides excellent support services with appropriate guidance and advice. The Association for Retarded Citizens (ARC) can provide similar services for the retarded child and his family. Parents' groups sponsored by these organizations talk about managing mental retardation or coping with cerebral palsy. They don't talk about seizures. Yet for parents of children who have intractable seizures, and where mental retardation and cerebral palsy frequently co-exist, the focus is often on seizures: "If only the seizures were controlled, it would be easier to deal with the other problems." It's important for you to decide what is really most important for your child. Maybe it is the seizures. But maybe it isn't. For some children the problems of mental retardation are far more important than the seizures themselves. For some children with cerebral palsy, mobility may be the principal problem. For parents of these children, UCP or the local ARC may provide the most important resources. If seizures are the central problem you may need to educate these organizations about epilepsy and about the special needs of children who have recurring seizures.

For children whose seizures are the dominant disability and mental retardation, for example, is of lower priority, at least for now, parents have often had difficulty finding help. There has been a gap in support services for the multiple handicapped child who also has seizures. Fortunately, the Epilepsy Foundation of America has recognized this need and, as part of its recommitment to serving *all* families, is in the process of developing new programs to meet this need.

The medical community also has failed to serve this population well. Developmental pediatricians trained to help manage the multiple problems of the disabled child and to help families find needed services frequently have less expertise in epilepsy than other conditions. Further, neurologists or epileptologists who do specialize in treating children's seizures often have inadequate expertise in managing family problems and in finding services. We need to develop better one-stop shopping for this comprehensive care. But until we do parents of a multi-handicapped child must continue to advocate and seek services with persistence and determination.

## Coping with Shattered Expectations

Parents of a newborn child have great expectations. These expectations are dashed when a child is diagnosed as having multiple severe handicaps. But such a diagnosis should not mean that expectations for your child must be abandoned. It means that your expectations must be modified, although your hopes may persist. Your expectations for your child need to be individualized. You should discuss them with your physician, but your doctor does not have a crystal ball. He may not be able to foresee with any great precision how well your child will be able to do.

Parents often tell us that their physician had said that their child would never walk and are angry that the doctor underestimated their child's abilities. Their child is now walking. Others are angry because their physician did not tell them that their child would have troubles in school or be retarded. When a child is only one, it may be difficult to predict how well he will talk, walk, or learn. When your child is three, your doctor may be able to be more precise in making predictions. By age eight, you and he will have a much better idea about learning problems. The more severely handicapped the child, the earlier accurate predictions can be made. *Betting on children is like betting on race horses; the more they've run, the better you will be able to predict their future success.*

Virtually no child stays the same forever. All children make progress. The rate of that progress is a measure of the severity of the neurologic damage. For the parents of a profoundly handicapped child, progress may be measured in terms of smiling, feeding, head control, or reaching—or even just an awareness that you are there. These milestones that parents of more normal children take for granted can be major achievements for profoundly handicapped children and their families. When your child is severely handicapped it may be difficult to hold great expectations for the future. Take pleasure in small accomplishments, deal with the bad things, and then set them aside. If you cope in small ways, day by day and week by week, coping will become easier.

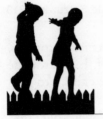

# 17. Epilepsy as a Psycho-social Disease

Epilepsy is usually considered a medical disorder. But for centuries it has been a psycho-social disease as well. This is not because of anything intrinsic to the disorder. Epilepsy is not confined to any social group, nor is it contagious. Epilepsy is a psycho-social disease because of the reactions, or perceived reactions, of society to persons with epilepsy, and because of the psychological and social problems often associated with the disorder.

Epilepsy is a chronic condition, but unlike most other chronic health conditions, which have constant problems, recurrent seizures of epilepsy wax and wane over time. Dr. William Lennox, considered one of the fathers of American epilepsy treatment, characterized the disorder as "a recurrent tidal wave" compared with the constant rough seas of many other chronic health disorders. This is an apt metaphor.

*Most* of the time, *most* people with epilepsy are normal, subject to the same stresses and strains as everyone else. *Most* of the time, seizures do not complicate their lives. Most individuals with epilepsy take their medication and go on. But then, usually without warning, some of these individuals with controlled epilepsy are suddenly swamped by the tidal wave of another seizure. After the seizure they usually right themselves and put their lives back in order, not knowing when, or if, another tidal wave will strike. Thus epilepsy is complicated by the uncertainty factor.

Where will your child fit on the broad spectrum of the epilepsies? Will he or she have "benign" epilepsy of childhood or one of the other chronic epilepsies in which recurrent seizures vary in frequency and severity? Will he have one of the additional disabilities sometimes associated with epilepsy?

The underpinnings of many future possible difficulties begin in childhood and are, to a large extent, the result of the psycho-social impact of epilepsy on the child and on the family. If the physician and the parent are sensitive to the possible development of these problems, many can be avoided.

## The Child's Self-perception

Self-image or self-esteem, as we have often said, is an important ingredient of success in later life. How does your child's self-image change after a seizure? The answer to this may depend on his self-image before the seizure. The change, if any, will depend on the type of seizure and its immediate effects on him, on his developmental age, and on what, if anything, follows the seizure. Most important, self-image and self-esteem will depend on how your child and the seizure are treated by you, by your friends and family, and by your doctor.

The response of family and friends is perhaps the principal determinant of the eventual outcome for the young child and the principal factor under your control for children of all ages.

Accurate and honest information appears an important ingredient of any child's self-perception, best documented for adolescents. In many studies, adolescents who were the least well-informed were the ones with the poorest psycho-social adjustment. Their adjustment did not correlate either with their seizure control or with their neurological normalcy. Adolescents who were most normal, who had no neurological abnormality, and whose seizures were under control often were most negative about their social adjustment because they were fearful about "being discovered." Those individuals who had a seizure in public were better able to adapt than those who still feared being "discovered." Children with epilepsy also had lower self-esteem, higher levels of anxiety, and feelings of less control than children with other health-related conditions.

Most of these problems can be prevented if your child is included in discussions of his epilepsy and its treatment. Age-appropriate discussion of epilepsy, of your child's particular type of seizures, and of the reason for taking medication is an important first step in an understanding and an acceptance of his condition. In one study, many children still believed they could swallow their tongues during a seizure. They feared that they might die. Unfounded apprehensions seem to be more damaging than the reality. Shielding your child from the facts to prevent him "from being scared" is more likely to lead to worse, but unspoken, fears than an honest and open discussion.

Your attitude toward your child and his seizures will affect his own. If you are frightened, he may be too, even if he doesn't understand why. If you are overprotective, he may respond by either becoming dependent or rebellious. Understanding that he is normal most of the time and honest calmness on your part will allow your child to get on with the process of developing independence and competence.

It should be the job of your physician and the team to assure that issues of honesty, overprotection, and dependency have been discussed with you and your spouse, and that you have come to terms with them. The epilepsy team should also discuss the seizures, medication, and reasonable restrictions with your child and make sure that you also have discussed them with him in age-appropriate terms.

Remember, ultimately epilepsy is your child's problem. If the seizures continue or if he must continue to take medication, then he will have to assume responsibility for his condition and its treatment. If your child is given a sense of control from the beginning, he will feel more responsible for his future life. We try to have these discussions with children when they are as young as five or six years of age. Responsibility clearly increases with age, but participation can rarely begin too early.

## Overprotection and Overindulgence

Overprotection often causes more handicap for a disabled child than the underlying health condition itself. Protection of their young is the natural reaction of parents. Even in the absence of disability, parents raising children must tread the fine line between protection and over-protection. This line changes with the age of the child and is challenged by the independent adult trying to emerge from the child during adolescence. Your natural reaction to protect your child is greatly magnified when he is injured. You naturally want to protect him from the cruelties of the public and his peers. You want to shield him from further physical and emotional injury. Your overprotection is magnified by your anxieties, fears, and often by an unwarranted sense of guilt. These are normal reactions, but they may deprive your child of the rewards of having tried and been successful.

❏ Roberta wanted to try out for cheerleading. It was very clear to her mother that her poorly controlled seizures and her general clumsiness would not allow her to make the squad. Rather than preventing her from competing, her mother helped Roberta to realize that many people try out but are unsuccessful and that while trying out was terrific, she needed to be able to cope with the possibility of not being selected. Her mother was there, taking lots of pictures. Indeed, Roberta did not make the squad, but she was thrilled to have been part of the process. She was not terribly disappointed with her failure and had some wonderful memories for her scrapbook.

Growing up requires risks to achieve benefits. Your child with epilepsy, like any child, needs opportunities to achieve independence. Opportunities necessarily entail risks. Think carefully about how much the epilepsy has really increased your child's risk.

The other side of overprotection is overindulgence. It can be equally destructive. "But if I yell at him, he might have a seizure." "He throws a tantrum when he doesn't get his own way, and I don't want to upset him." "She's been through so much, I don't want to keep her from. . . ." We hear these types of statements from many parents. When the seizures are subsequently brought under control with medication, these parents are left with a miserable, spoiled, undisciplined child or adolescent who is not handicapped by epilepsy but socially handicapped in other ways.

## Attitudes of Brothers and Sisters

Sibling love, as well as sibling rivalry, is normal. The reaction of your child's brother or sister to a sibling with epilepsy will depend on age and developmental stage, but most of all on your reaction to epilepsy and to your children.

All children fantasize, and it is not uncommon for a sibling to believe that he caused his brother's seizures by playing roughly or pushing and causing his brother to fall. Children often wish for things to happen to their brother or sister. If something happens, then guilt is a common response. These feelings may be compounded by jealousy because you are giving too much attention to the child who has seizures. Brothers or sisters may show these feelings by "acting out," by withdrawing, or by signs of depression, any of which may affect school performance and sleep patterns.

Children often believe also that epilepsy, like measles, is contagious and that they might catch it, too. This fear should be discussed openly within the family.

Your other children may be drawn into a pattern of overprotection or overindulgence. Either you or they may say, "Don't play so roughly, you might bring on a seizure." "Don't let him get so excited." "Give him the toy, or he'll get upset and have a seizure." Such statements give enormous leverage to your child to manipulate his environment.

Most of these problems can be avoided by your sensitivity to the effects of your child's epilepsy on his brothers and sisters and openness and honesty about your own feelings about the epilepsy and your continued love for all of your children. It is important that you initiate discussions with your other children and that no matter how time-consuming and preoccupying your child's seizure problems may be, you find some time to spend individually with the others, talking and doing something special with them and for them.

Studies have shown that, while there is always an impact on siblings whose brother or sister has a disability, if handled appropriately, that impact is positive. Brothers and sisters can become stronger, more sympathetic, more empathetic, and more caring adults.

## Attitudes of Friends

It is up to you and your child to tell friends about the epilepsy. The information conveyed, and the persons to whom it is conveyed, should depend on the type and frequency of the seizures. For the child with absence or partial complex seizures that occur with some frequency, it is far better for the friend to understand the seizures than to assume that the child is "weird," on drugs, or going crazy. One of our teenagers with unrecognized absence seizures had been nicknamed "Spacey" by her friends. It is more useful for a friend to understand what to do should a seizure occur and not to panic.

Unless the seizures are frequent, it is unnecessary to inform everyone with whom your child comes in contact. However, his good friends and families with whom he spends time should be aware of his seizures and how they are controlled. In general, the fears and apprehensions that are consequences of ignorance are far worse than any reality.

"Should I tell my date?" is a question we are often asked by teenagers. Again, this depends on the frequency and type of the seizures. Certainly if a relationship begins to become serious, your teenager should be self-confident enough to talk openly about his or her condition.

### How Common Are Psycho-social Problems?

It is hard to tell how common such problems are, since there are biases in all studies. Children with psycho-social problems are far more likely to be identified and included in studies than those without problems. Also, children with continuing seizures are more likely to be identified than the 80 percent whose seizures are completely controlled or outgrown.

Whatever the true incidence, such problems are sufficiently common that they should be monitored. Problems with learning and even with retardation are usually caused by brain injury rather than the seizures themselves. Learning problems, as well as hyperactivity and behavioral problems, may be caused by medication. Close monitoring of your child's school performance should be your responsibility and if you have concerns, you should discuss them with your physician.

Depression is not uncommon in children. It may be hard to identify. Symptoms of depression include sleep disturbances, school problems, fatigue or listlessness, lack of enthusiasm, easy crying, and irritability, among others. Depression can be due to medication, particularly phenobarbital. But depression also may be a consequence of a child's or family's reaction to the seizures and their treatment. If you are concerned about these problems, you should discuss them with your doctor. Early identification of depression can lead to earlier help.

*In general, psycho-social problems are sufficiently common in children with epilepsy that families and physicians should be alert to them. Preventive discussions with members of the family and the school may avoid problems and permit early identification. Psycho-social problems should not be allowed to become a handicap.*

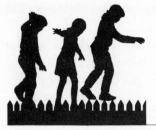

# 18. Counseling:
# A Dialogue

Guidance and counseling, commonly used as synonymous terms, have somewhat different connotations to us. Guidance is something one person provides to another. It implies, to us at least, something actively given and passively received. Counseling, on the other hand, implies something done together and requires active participation by both parties. We believe this distinction is important.

Physicians often speak of patients as compliant or non-compliant, meaning they have or haven't followed their instructions. Implied in the word compliant is a sense of submissiveness. We often assume that a person with seizures should do exactly what we tell them to. We forget that it is the patient who experiences the seizures, who is encumbered by the stigma of epilepsy, and who may experience side effects from medication we prescribe. We forget that the disorder is the patient's and, therefore, that the patient must ultimately exercise his own control. However, in a more positive sense, compliance is not submissiveness but reflects a partnership in which the patient agrees with a therapy we recommend and will follow it.

If the patient or, in the case of young children, the family is to exercise the control, then they must be educated to become active partners in the decision-making processes. They must be informed about their condition or their child's condition and about the likely future. The patient—or the parents of a young child—must assume the responsibility for that future. They must determine their own goals and aspirations. Some use terms like "owning your own disease" or "empowering the consumer."

We prefer to talk in terms of a partnership and counseling. Then the physician and his team are in the more appropriate position of teachers, counselors, and supporters on this road to seizure control and to medical as well as psycho-social well-being.

## "Who Needs Counseling?"

"I believe that everyone touched by epilepsy needs education and information. Each should understand the medical information about epilepsy and the social ramifications of the disorder. But many have a difficult time coming to terms with the diagnosis of 'epilepsy,' whether for themselves or for their child. For most, the diagnosis is overwhelming. The enormous amount of information initially given is hard for parents and children to comprehend. Often they find it difficult to stand back from the immediate situation and achieve a perspective. A counselor may be able to help them sift through the information the physician has provided, to explain it again, perhaps in different terms, and then to help them begin working on a process of coping. Parents, often numbed by the initial diagnosis and overwhelming amount of information, worry that in the numbness they appear unable to comprehend, unable even to think of appropriate questions. Parents voice concern that the doctor may think they are stupid. A counselor can step in when this numbness subsides and help them voice the questions they were too stunned to ask before.

"In working with people who have epilepsy, the counselor has to develop trust. In developing that trust, the most important ingredient is total honesty. I emphasize to them that I am speaking to them as a counselor, not as a person who knows what it is like to have a seizure, since I've never had one. I tell them that I don't walk in their shoes but that what I offer are some tools, developed by working with lots of people, the tools which they need to deal with their epilepsy so that it does not take over their lives.

"What most people want is some control over their lives. What I want for every person with epilepsy is for them to have ownership and control over their seizure disorder. A counselor can't give them complete control over the medical aspects of their disorder but can help them to gain the best control possible over their seizures. She can help them gain control over the social ramifications of epilepsy and of their own self-image.

"A referral for counseling can come from the family itself, recognizing their own need for help; it may come from the physician or anyone in contact with the child or family who recognizes that they need additional help in understanding or coping.

"Many people have their own way of coping and do very nicely. But often when the family is under stress things can just come apart. Sometimes the stresses are due to misperceived guilt or an effort to fix blame; sometimes fears or jealousy among siblings are the cause; occasionally, people who seem to be coping well just get tired of pretending that everything is OK, that nothing has changed. They need to unload and say, 'I'm sick of pretending that I'm coping well. My child is sick of pretending that everything is still fine in school.' This pretending that everything is OK may work for awhile, but is useful only until acceptance of the epilepsy and of its problems ultimately occurs. These are some of the things that bring a person or family in for counseling.

"Counseling should be part of the initial educational process, not just directed at working out later problems. Preventive counseling should begin, then, at the time of the diagnosis. If the patient and the family don't understand that treatment will require trial-and-error medication adjustment, they may lose trust in their doctor when other seizures occur. They will often feel that the doctor hasn't fixed the epilepsy. If the patient has side effects of the medication and has not been made aware of that possibility, they may feel the medicine is no good rather than considering that it needs to be adjusted. Children or adolescents who never seen a seizure will have trouble understanding their friends' reactions when a seizure occurs or the fear that others may have of a seizure's occurring. If the family hasn't been warned about the dangers and consequences of overprotection, then they naturally overprotect their child and have to suffer the consequences later.

"Counseling is not for everyone. Some don't need it, and some don't want it. If a person or a family doesn't want it, then it will be of no use to them. All you can do is leave the door open for them to come back later. Another possibility is to try to connect a family with another family or a support group that may be less threatening.

"Sometimes counseling is crisis intervention; something catastrophic has happened and the individual needs to talk about it. Sometimes families just need help or further discussion in order to understand better the information the physician has given them. But sometimes intervening in those crises or rediscussing the interpretation of the information uncovers a whole can of worms. Suddenly the counselor finds other underlying stresses in the family that need to be addressed. Families who are dealing with epilepsy are just like other families with all their stresses and tensions. Epilepsy is an additional stress, one that can exacerbate and expose all of the others.

"All families need to be able to communicate, and a counselor gives both the individual and the family an opportunity to do just that. They need to talk about the epilepsy but also to talk about all of the other things which affect families, things like expectations, fears, responsibilities, restrictions, and feelings about themselves and others.

"Counseling and education should involve the child, even the child as young as five or six. It is a disservice to leave them out. Involving them early begins the process of ownership of their condition which, over the long run, is so important in helping them to cope.

"The counselor doesn't cope for them. The child, the teenager, the adult, the family will have to cope for themselves. All I'm there to do is to be the catalyst, to give them the tools to achieve the benefits of confidence and independence."

## Where Counseling Helps: An Example

❑ "Karen is one of the best examples of the importance of counseling. Karen had her first seizure when she was about ten. It was a tonic-clonic seizure, and then she had a few complex partial seizures later. Medication controlled these for about two years, but when she was about twelve she again began having seizures and first came to Hopkins. The doctor wanted to change Karen's medicine but was also very concerned about the fact that things were going poorly for her in school and thought the cause might be a problem with the school's acceptance of her seizures. The doctor asked me to see Karen and find out what was going on.

"Karen was a very shy young lady, and during our first visit all she did was cry. I couldn't get her to talk at all. So I asked her to keep a journal, to go home and write down her thoughts about everything she felt, so that when she came back we could talk about them. What we discovered was that the problems weren't in school, they were at home. The major problem was a father who blamed Karen for all of the family strife, arguing, and financial problems.

Eventually we asked her family to come in to talk. Her father never would participate. He was a very domineering type, her mother a rather meek lady. The counseling, which went on weekly for over a year, helped Karen gain control and do better in school. This may have had less to do with understanding epilepsy than with the fact that the family situation changed. Her mother, who ostensibly came to counseling to understand more about epilepsy, gained insight into her own problems. She ultimately decided to divorce Karen's father. This led to an additional need for family counseling as they readjusted to a single-parent family.

"It took a long time for Karen to realize that the problems were really not due to her but to the dynamics of her family. She finally realized that she was not responsible for having epilepsy. She learned that her medical bills were not the cause of the family's financial problems. She eventually saw that her father was just using the epilepsy as an excuse and that she was suffering from his blame and her own feelings of guilt."

*"So what you're saying is that the epilepsy wasn't Karen's problem, is that right?"*

"Well, not exactly. Karen's seizures were not a major problem, but she had no education about epilepsy. She was surrounded by all of these family arguments and strife, and she said to herself, 'Hey, I'm the only one who is sick. I'm the only one who is different. Therefore, all of this must be my fault.' This also led to her doing poorly in school, which made her think that she was dumb, which she attributed to her epilepsy. All of these things contributed to a terrible self-image. So we had to work on these issues. We also had to work with her brother and sister, who were jealous that she was getting a disproportionate share of attention. They needed to see that Karen was the victim not the cause of parental discord.

"Helping Karen took a year. We would reexamine the thoughts she recorded in her journal. I challenged her to do things. At the start, she was tired all the time, had no energy, wanted only to sleep. We wondered if this was medication, but it probably was depression. Karen enjoyed athletics but had given them up because of her epilepsy and her school problems. We got her involved in just one sport and watched her energy level increase. When she found she could participate despite her epilepsy, things began to go better.

"Initially Karen was having seizures every few months. With medication adjustment (and as she got older) she would go for almost a year without a seizure. It seemed as if she'd almost made it; our state then required a person to be seizure-free for one year to get a driver's license. The rug was pulled out from under her each time. But, through counseling, she had become a stronger person and was able to deal with the recurrence of seizures. With each recurrence she was, of course, disappointed and angry, but most of all she was determined. Most of those recurrences happened when she had tested the limits of how little sleep she could exist on, of how much she could drink, or of how long she could miss her medication. Gradually she learned those limits and that the seizures and the driving were under her control. With each of these recurrences, she would come back to see the doctor and to see me. She would be angry and extremely upset, but I could support her. I never made light of her problems, and that is very important. What may seem to be small problems to the counselor and possibly to the parents can be big problems to the teenager."

## "How Do You Help Teenagers Cope?"

"Well, what else are they going to do? I ask teenagers, 'What are your choices?' They could go in their rooms, close the door, and never come out again. That would be a choice. If you help people discover alternatives and allow them to make their own choices, eventually they can find the best way to deal with their problems. There really isn't anything to do but to pick yourself up and go on, is there?

"But sometimes things don't go so well. People with epilepsy have to walk a fine line between hope and reality. Life is not always fair, but what are they going to do about it? You just have to deal with it. Counseling often can be very helpful in enabling people to see that.

"I saw Karen every week or two at the beginning, but later, as things got better, our meetings would be less frequent. She would call just to let me know how things were going or if there was a problem. We got through her first date (she learned that girls with epilepsy could date and be attractive, like everyone else). We discussed who you tell about your epilepsy and when. She didn't tell every date, but when she began to be serious about one person she made certain that he knew about her seizures. She told her close friends and also the coach of her team.

"Now Karen is in college. She first went to junior college to prove to her father that she could do it, and then he agreed to let her transfer out-of-state. She is doing very well. She now has a good self-image. Her seizures are under control, although there is still an occasional seizure when she tests the limits."

**"How do you respond then?"**

"I just say, 'Hey, you've got to pay the piper. You know the rules and what you can do. It's your choice.' Teenagers want to be in control. Like all other children and adolescents, there is a need to test limits, to explore. That is a time-tested way of growing. It's no different for kids with epilepsy; but they have additional boundaries to test. They don't like parents or anyone else telling them what to do. They don't like having to take medication, because it doesn't seem to be under their control. As Karen has become more mature, she really understands. She knows it *is* her choice whether she takes medicine and how she treats her body. That gives her control.

"Another thing which has been a big help for Karen's self-image is that she has become a counselor to other teenagers. We have asked her to participate in conferences for parents and others. On occasion, we have asked her to talk with younger teens, either individually or in groups. She is a role model, and that works out well for everyone."

**"Is there much difference between counseling teenagers and counseling adults with epilepsy?"**

"I work mostly with children and teens, so I'm more likely to talk about them, but I counsel adults as well. Every person is an individual. Some are more mature than others. Sure, teens have their own hang-ups and you need to help them achieve independence and get over the hump from child to adult. While there are many similarities in counseling adults, it is sometimes more difficult, especially if they've had seizures since childhood. Too frequently, adequate counseling and education were not available to them. They've spent so many years with a poor self-image; reconstructing is more difficult than building it right in the first place. They need to learn how to take control of their epilepsy and also of their lives. That's one of the reasons why I feel so strongly that children need to take ownership of their seizures at the earliest possible point."

**"Does counseling always work out this well?"**

"Not for everyone, but it does for many. Sometimes you have to take different approaches. The clinic had one teenage boy whose seizures were under complete control for long periods of time, and then he would have another tonic-clonic seizure. He swore that he took his medicine, but at the time of each seizure the blood levels would be low. He was never interested in counseling. He thought he was too macho and that he could handle it. He was really a good kid, off at college, and he wanted to get his own car. In Maryland you now can drive when you have been seizure-free for three months. Finally, after he wrecked the family car in what was presumed to be a seizure, the doctor said to him, 'Look, you are wasting my time and your parents' money. I don't care if you have seizures or if you never drive. I don't want to see you again until you can look me in the eye and tell me that you have been taking the medicine regularly and not drinking. If you have a seizure under those circumstances and the blood level is good, then I'll work hard with you to get the seizures under control. Then perhaps we'll try another medication, but not until that time. What's more, I'd suggest to your parents that they not let you drive until you've shown that you can take responsibility.'"

"The doctor told this to the boy and then told this to the parents in the boy's presence. John has not had any seizures since. Sometimes tough love is necessary, and putting the responsibility in the patient's court gives a person the control that is needed. It's their epilepsy, not their parents, not the physician's, not the counselor's.

"This concept of control can apply to other issues as well. We recently saw a teenage girl who had not had seizures for two years. We suggested that she begin to taper the medication now, in advance of starting to drive. She wanted to be off medication, but was afraid she would have another seizure and, worst of all, that she might have one at school. We talked about her fears, but we left the decision about stopping the medicine to her. Several months later she decided to try it, and has done well. These were things she wouldn't discuss with the doctor, but would discuss with me. I seemed to her to be less threatening."

## Counseling the Younger Child

"Whether counseling a younger child is different from counseling a teenager depends on the age of the child, the child's level of understanding, and the child's problems. Let me tell you about Jenny, who was nine years old when I first met her. She was a bright youngster, one of four children. Her mother was a former nurse and had a fair amount of medical knowledge about epilepsy. The father had gone back to law school at night, so the family was under real financial stress. In addition to caring for the family, her mom was working two jobs. Let me tell you, tensions in that family were real high.

"Jenny had several seizures, but that wasn't the reason she was referred to us. She was initially referred because her doctor thought she might have a degenerative brain disease. Over the previous year, she had deteriorated dramatically, both at school and at home. She was always sick with headaches or stomach aches and was missing a fair amount of school. Visits to the doctor's office weren't helping the family financial problems, either. Neither her mother nor her physician could tell what was related to the seizures or to the medication or what was psychological. She had become a very belligerent and disruptive child, causing havoc in the family. Her actual seizures were not that bad, but the family was disintegrating, even though they wanted to stay together.

"Jenny's behavior was the main issue at our first meeting. She didn't like taking medicine. She didn't like being sick and going to the doctors. All kids seek attention, but some do not distinguish between attention for the positive things they do and attention for misbehaving. Jenny was not always aware of what she was doing. Her temper outbursts and not feeling well took up much of the limited time this family had for each other. Her brother and sister resented all the attention and concern Jen was getting, and they let her know it; they also began to manifest the same symptoms in attempts to draw attention to themselves. The family was a mess. This is a good example of how epilepsy becomes a family problem, not just a problem for the affected individual.

"Jenny, although only nine, had many long-range questions: 'Do big girls have these seizures? Can they have babies?' Things like that. I arranged for Karen to have lunch with us. And the two just talked. They talked about seizures, about medication, about boys. What Karen provided for her was something I couldn't provide; she was the role model Jenny needed. Actually, it was as good for Karen as for Jen; it provided Karen with a sense of self-esteem, a sense of helping.

"You know, out of this counseling come many good things, and sometimes it takes awhile to see all of them. Another young lady who had a rough time as a teenager, both with her very frequent mixed seizures and with an overprotective father, is now married and has a baby. The family recently had a real scare when they thought she had cancer. They really panicked, but Greta remained cool. She handled it far better than her folks. The diagnosis proved wrong, and when we talked about it recently she said, 'You know, I went through so much in learning to deal with my epilepsy that it made me a much stronger individual.'

"One of the best things about this job is the friends you make with the kids. They'll call you up years later, as Greta did, just to say 'Hi!' or to tell you they're engaged, whatever. They've become my friends.

"There's another child I want to tell you about. Remember Jeb? He was only six. He had the mildest of seizures, just a few absence seizures, and he was adorable. But what an anxious family. Mom, a former nurse, read everything available and learned of allergic reactions to medication the doctors had never seen before. Jeb was having some stomach problems and had become a monster at home. His mother thought he was not doing well in school. He had taken to fighting at school and misbehaving at home. Jeb was very verbal, bright, and with lots of questions. Both the doctors and I took him aside and explained his epilepsy. We asked him to write down his questions and asked his sister, who was a year younger, to have her mother list hers. We promised to discuss them at the next visit. Jeb knew the family was very upset, but he didn't know why. He felt different and asked, 'What's wrong with me?' His mom was extremely knowledgeable, but even though she was a former nurse, she was really just a mom. She couldn't step back, and so she became very nervous. She called me every day for several weeks. That's another way to do counseling, just to provide reassurance by phone.

"Jeb also was given permission to call me. He didn't always need to have his mom interpreting things for him. He could tell me, 'I don't like this,' 'I'm sick of that.' 'Do you want to know how I did in school today?'

"What he did was to take ownership of his condition, his medication, and of his young life. That's pretty remarkable for a six-year-old and also remarkable for a parent to permit it and still provide appropriate supervision.

"His sister, who also played an important role, had her own questions. Her first question was 'Will I catch this?' That is a typical question I hear from brothers and sisters. Her second question was, 'Why did this happen to Jeb?' Only after she knew that she was safe could her concern for her brother come out. There were other questions, 'Do more boys than girls get epilepsy?' The questions themselves were less important than the fact that both children had the right to ask them. Each child was important, and both were an important part of Jeb's getting well.

"Too often doctors and even counselors get caught up with the parents' concerns about their child's epilepsy and the child's own concerns about his seizures. We forget the brothers and sisters. Epilepsy is a family problem. It touches everybody. It's important to let brothers and sisters express their concerns. It's important to help them to ask questions that they can't articulate easily. In our experience virtually every brother or sister has fears, misunderstandings, and resentments. It's imperative that they talk about them and be part of the family's acceptance of epilepsy.

"When it was time to discontinue medication, Jeb was the one who was allowed to make the final decision. It was discussed with him and his mom. He went home to think about it and discuss it with the family. Even at seven, he understood that there was a risk of having more seizures and that he might have to restart medicine. I strongly believe that it is important to be honest with people, especially with children.

"When he was scheduled to come back and tell us his decision, I was out of town, so Jeb changed his appointment because he wanted me to be there, too. He said that I was a part of all of this, and he wanted me to hear his decision.

*"I guess the important thing I want people to understand about counseling is that it is not a routine thing. It has to be individualized for each child, for each adult, for each family, and for each problem. Education about epilepsy underlies much of it, but understanding kids and family dynamics is probably the largest part. There is also a large element of common sense."*

## When Counseling Didn't Help

*"You've only told us about your successes. Tell us about your failures. Everybody with epilepsy doesn't end up happy, having outgrown epilepsy and off in college, do they?"*

"No. One of the distressing facts you have to face as a counselor is that you can't save the world. There are some pathetic people out there. Yes, there are some sad kids, and some miserable parents, as well. There are some who enjoy being unhappy. There are some who derive their pleasures from saying 'poor me.' There are those who just don't have any motivation, and some who don't have enough motivation to change at the time you see them. You have to try to keep communications open, so if their motivation develops later, they can come back and get help.

"The successes I've been talking about are primarily among the 80 percent of children whose seizures can be brought under control and who don't have other handicaps. In this group it is easier to give them hope. You can easily and honestly say to them, 'Look, most people like you will have their seizures completely controlled. You will probably outgrow your epilepsy.' I can give them some positives to look forward to.

"For the families who have a retarded child with epilepsy, or with cerebral palsy and epilepsy, or a child with some other combination of multiple handicaps, then you may have to define success and failure differently. We often are faced with families with a severely-damaged child who also has seizures. They come to us before they really recognize how damaged the child is and how limited that child will be. The parents will focus on the seizures and the medication and overlook the other underlying problems.

"Parents like this will need a lot of support over a long period of time. You can't just tell them right off, 'Hey, your child is never going to walk or talk or do anything.' It is important to give them hope. Everyone needs to maintain some hope. But you have to help them to become realistic, gradually to come to terms with the child's problems and to accept them. Realistic acceptance, coupled with hope, is the goal I set for these parents.

"You have to help them to see and appreciate the small successes every child achieves. These little successes—smiling, responding, turning over, making a sound—may be minimal achievements to you, but they are major achievements to the parent who has waited for them so long. Parents' reactions to severely-handicapped children like these often will depend on ethnic background and on the social context in which they were raised. There is also a lot of individual variation. It is amazing the reserves of strength that reside deep in many people.

"I don't know how I would respond if I were thrust into the situation that faces many of these parents. And I don't think anyone knows how he will respond until he actually has to face it. But, somehow, virtually all of them do respond in a positive fashion. Somehow, virtually all of them learn to cope.

"What they require most of all is support. They need to realize that they aren't the only ones who have faced a tragedy. They need support from husband or wife, from grandparents, and from friends. The counselor can be a major source of that support but must also help in finding other community and family sources. I try to make sure that the grandparents are educated about the epilepsy and about the child's other problems; if grandparents do not understand, they can be very destructive instead of supportive of the family.

"In many cases fathers are more fortunate than the mothers who are at home because they don't have to live with the problem twenty-four hours a day. They go to work and have other distractions and other responsibilities. Too frequently the burden (and it can be a burden) falls on the mother, and that's not fair. One of my jobs is to try to make sure that the father stays involved, that he comes in for the counseling sessions, and that he shares some of the burden. I don't mean just the physical care of the child. He must shoulder some of the emotional burden, as well. Men often handle grief in a different fashion from women. They can bury themselves in their work and avoid having to face their grief and their emotions. This is less common with women, who seem to take on the responsibility, even when it grinds them down. They have to face the problems hourly, without a refuge. Working women can have an even worse problem. Rather than using work as a refuge, work becomes an additional responsibility. They still have the child and the problem back home. We find that many parents don't share these problems very well. They need help in communicating with each other, and in learning to share the burdens. It is important to try to keep the lines of communication open between the husband and wife. It is surprising how often they just don't talk. It is essential that the wife get some relief from her role, even if it is just an hour or two to go out to the market without the child, to go shopping on a Saturday when the husband is off work, to go away for a weekend or to a movie and dinner. A brief respite can make things more tolerable.

"When there are other children, it is critical that each gets a share of the parents' insufficient time. Each child should be made to feel special for a period of time, however brief. They should be taken out, played with, anything which is special for them, so they feel they still count. Parents need to realize that this handicapped child, who could consume thirty-six hours of every day, is not the only one who is important in the family.

"It is important for you as parents to understand that it is all right to be angry—angry at the doctors, at the system, at society-at-large. It's all right to be angry at the child, even when you know it is not his fault. These are normal feelings, and you're not a bad mother or father for feeling them. But you can't let the anger be the controlling force in your life. You have to learn to keep it in its place. Just as I tell some of the teenagers, 'Hey, life is unfair, but what are you going to do? What are your choices?' when you explore your choices you realize that they are very limited. You can't give the child back, although there are times when you might wish you could. There may even be times when you wish your child was dead, but he isn't. These thoughts are not incompatible with your basic love for your child. It's hard to put your child in an institution, even if you want to. Usually you're trapped.

"It's my job to help you find and use whatever resources are available. Solutions to some problems are obvious, but it's hard for families to think of everything on their own. I've usually heard the problem before. It's much easier for me to make suggestions about what you can do and where you can go for help. The work and follow-up is up to you.

"Some of the new, state-run pre-school early-intervention programs like Child Find are helpful in getting the parents of handicapped children, and the infant or young child himself, involved with appropriate stimulation and physical therapy. Schools now are taking these handicapped children at a young age, at least for part of the day. These programs give the parents some hope, some respite, and more realistic expectations about their child's progress and future.

"While counseling is fun and rewarding when you're dealing with a teenager like Karen (who you know will be a winner if only she'll get her act together), at times counseling can be even more challenging and more rewarding when you have a family with a severely-damaged child. Just think what you have accomplished when you help them to cope, to grow with the situation, to make the best of it, whatever that is, for themselves and for their child. If you look at the alternatives, such as the family breaking up, then you will have a single parent facing that future alone. Or the child could end up in a foster home with the family disintegrated. If you look at these bleak alternatives, then anything you can do to help the family to cope and to make a reasonable life for themselves and for their child is a success. If you define success in these terms, yes, we are usually, but not always, successful."

## Acceptance: The Biggest Problem

*"What do you find is the biggest problem for parents of multiply handicapped children?"*

"There's little question in my mind that the biggest hurdle is acceptance of the child. I don't mean that the parents don't love him or her right from the start. They do! They love the child, but they also love the image of the child that they carry in their minds. As I said before, none of us knows how we will cope with a child who doesn't meet our expectations. Even those who have had contact with handicapped children, who say they could cope, don't really know. Everyone has to go through the stages of grieving for the child who isn't as you planned, forgetting the child who is the image in your mind, before you can reach the stage of acceptance. For some parents, this can take a long time. But gradually people come to the realization of what their child can and can't do. You have to wait for the parents to come to those realizations themselves. They don't listen if you just tell them. You can help them to see, but, ultimately, they have to see for themselves before they can accept.

"In the meantime, the counselor has to be supportive. It's important to praise parents for what they are doing and to reassure them that they are doing everything possible. It is important to nurture their hope, but to try to temper that hope slowly with realism. It's a long, tough process for both the parents and for the counselor. But in the long run it's worth it."

*"What do you recommend parents do about friends who seem so uncomfortable around them?"*

"Friends, even good friends, may be uncomfortable asking about your child's problems. They may be so uncomfortable they can't even ask how he's doing, or what's new? In many, perhaps most cases, it's not because they don't care. Perhaps it's because they care too much and are afraid of hurting your feelings or bringing you more pain. Perhaps the best way for you to help them is to bring the questions up. Make them feel that you are comfortable talking about your child and his problems with them. You may have to be the one to take the lead."

### *"What about the handicapped young adult?"*

"One of the saddest experiences for a counselor is to encounter a young adult with limitations, whose seizures are under control but who has been so overprotected by loving and caring parents that as a child he never learned to care for himself, never learned survival skills. The parents are now getting older and finally realize they won't be around forever to care for him. They begin to worry about what will happen.

"Our local epilepsy association has apartments where we teach these individuals independent living and survival skills. But the skills are much harder to teach and to learn at an older age. It is difficult to break patterns of dependency that have built up over the years. Much of the overprotection and the resultant handicap could have been prevented if the family and the child had had good early counseling. The life of the whole family would have been much better."

### *"Is there anything else you'd like to emphasize?"*

"There are a couple of things that I would like to emphasize. First, people, particularly parents, have to remember that kids with epilepsy are kids first. You can't ascribe all of their problems to epilepsy. Kids fight, they sulk, they rebel, they don't do their chores. Epilepsy is not responsible for all of the child's problems. Epilepsy can influence and increase the magnitude of the problems. But how the child handles the epilepsy and how the parents handle both epilepsy and the child will influence that child's future. Much of the counseling I do is the same counseling I would do for any parent of any child who had some problems. I have to help the child and the family deal with the problems in the context of the epilepsy and how everyone has reacted to it.

"Another thing I find useful is contracts. My part of the contract is to be open, honest, and available. The other person's part depends on the goals and on the person's age. A reward system is always useful, independent of age. Setting small goals which can be achieved is very important. For children, it may be little things like brushing teeth, making their beds, doing one chore. These chores give children an area in which to succeed; they get their reward, and slowly they learn to take responsibility. When the child demonstrates responsibility in one area, then we can begin to work on another. Perhaps they are then ready to begin to assume responsibility for remembering to take their own medication, without the parent reminding, or giving the medication. This is then the child's first step in assuming control over seizures and over his or her own life.

"For adolescents, it may be something in school or small things at home: washing the dishes, cleaning their room. For adults it would be a different goal, but something they clearly could achieve and for which they would receive a reward, even if the reward was just winning my praise. Gradually they learn to take control and to assume responsibility, and ultimately that responsibility is extended to their epilepsy. I don't think there is any more rewarding job than helping these children and their families achieve their full potential.

"I've certainly seen good counseling done by nurses, psychologists, social workers, psychiatrists, and doubtless many others. But I've also seen well-trained counselors who may be excellent with other types of problems but who feel uncomfortable working with kids or with adults who have epilepsy. To be a good epilepsy counselor, a deep knowledge about epilepsy and how it affects people is important. Many counselors are just not sufficiently familiar with seizures and their effects and so are unable to help families become comfortable and cope. Sometimes the personalities of the counselor and the parent or child do not mesh. If working with one counselor is unsuccessful, try another. Counselors must remember that, unlike other handicapping conditions, epilepsy is not present all the time. It is not a visible handicap. It's not like cerebral palsy or mental retardation. You have to help the kids and the families to cope in a different fashion, with an episodic condition.

"Before we stop, I want to emphasize again the words *control, self-image,* and *ownership.* Everyone wants control. You have to help children and adolescents with epilepsy to take control. You can't do it for them. It's not the counselor's epilepsy. It's not *my* problem. They have to do the work. It's their choice. They have to develop their self-image, and giving them small things at which they can succeed is a first step. They have to develop the self-image before they can achieve the control.

"You know, what keeps me doing this is that the rewards are so great. Can you imagine how it feels to have people like Jenny's family tell me that they would not be a whole family if I hadn't been there? That's pretty big stuff. And the kids—you've become a part of their lives. While you may not need to continue to see them or counsel them, they'll just call you up to touch base and let you know how things are going. It's hard to beat that feeling."

**Part Five**
# Living with Epilepsy

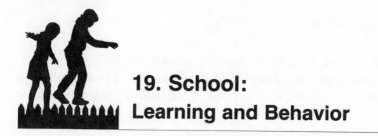

# 19. School:
# Learning and Behavior

*"Will my child have problems in school?"*

*"Are my child's school problems due to his epilepsy?"*

There are no easy answers to these questions, since no one has a crystal ball to see how your child will do in the future. Even if your child is having school problems, your physician can't make a blanket statement that the child's school problems are or are not due to epilepsy. Answers to questions such as these require much more information.

Why does one child do well in school? Why does another have school problems? A child's "doing well in school" and "school problems" depend, in part, on his intelligence, on whether he has a learning disability, on his attitude towards school and about himself, and on the teacher's and the school's attitudes toward him and toward epilepsy. Let us reassure you first that:

• There is NO reason to worry about the possibility of school problems, unless your child is encountering and demonstrating problems.
• Most children with epilepsy do well in school.
• Most children with epilepsy DO NOT have learning problems or social problems in school.
• There IS reason to be aware that school problems could occur, since they do occur more frequently in children who have epilepsy.

You should also remember that lots of children without epilepsy have problems of various kinds in school. Thus, even if your child does have problems in school, they may not be related to epilepsy itself.

## Intelligence

Most children have "normal" intelligence; the "average" IQ is given the number 100, and 95 percent of children have IQs from 70 to 130. While there are many questions and much debate about the meaning of an IQ score and about the tests by which it is determined, in a rough way it is shorthand for how a child will function in school. Most children with epilepsy have IQ scores within this normal range. However, if psychologists look at the range and distribution of the IQ scores for a large number of children with epilepsy, they find a larger than expected number with scores in the low-normal range. This is not because of the epilepsy itself, but usually because of what has caused the epilepsy. If the child had meningitis or brain damage, or problems with the brain's development, then those problems could have both affected the child's intelligence and have caused the epilepsy.

Intelligence is the result of many factors. The intelligence of parents and the environment in which the child is raised are the most important. Thus, one factor to consider, if your child is having difficulties in school, is his IQ. If his IQ is toward the lower end of the normal range, learning to read or doing math may be more difficult for him than for the rest of the class. The frustration associated with these difficulties could cause behavior problems and "acting out." Since these problems might be easily solved by a different class placement or by special help, it is important to recognize their cause early. Knowledge of the child's intelligence might also change your expectations and those of his teachers, removing undue pressure.

A very bright child, in a class that is beneath her abilities, may also be bored and not do the work or might act out. So occasionally a child's school problems are because the child is too smart for the class and requires more challenge.

One wonderful first grader was referred to us by his teacher because he was having difficulties reading and was not participating in class. She wanted him tested for neurologic dysfunction. His parents couldn't understand since he had no reading problems at home, only at school. A few questions to his family revealed that his favorite activity at home was reading *Popular Mechanics* and trying to build some of the things he found there. His response to the school problem was, "I'm not going to read about Dick and Jane and Spot. They're for babies." This young man clearly did not have a reading problem or a learning problem, he had a classroom problem.

Medications may also affect the child's performance in school and on IQ tests.

## Learning Problems

Intelligence is only one of the critical factors in the child's ability to learn. There can be other problems. For example, reading is a complex task. The child must first see the letters and the seeing must then be translated into electrical signals in the eye. These signals are then sent to the occipital lobe of the brain. From there the message goes to the association areas of the brain in the parietal lobe where the symbols are interpreted. Meaning comes from association with something that the child remembers, memories which must be retrieved from the frontal and temporal lobes.

Thus problems with reading could occur at many levels. A child with visual problems who needs glasses may not be able to see the letters. A child with damage in the occipital lobes might have normal eyes but might not "see" the letters. One with damage in the association areas of the brain might be able to see the letters but might not be able to recognize them. Problems in other areas might keep him from being able to retrieve the memories that give the words meaning. These varied difficulties with reading often go under the heading of "dyslexia." "Dys-" means not working properly, and "lexia" means having to do with words. In most children the basic cause of the dyslexia is not understood. There clearly is a higher incidence of this type of learning problem in children with epilepsy.

Learning by listening is also a multi-stage process. It involves hearing and paying attention to what is said. It involves transmission of the electrical signals to the association cortex where they must be recognized and associated with memories and actions. Thus, another type of learning problem might be associated with problems in hearing, attending, word recognition, and the association of words with memories.

These are but two of the many multi-step processes that may cause a child to have difficulties with learning. It is rare for anyone to be completely abnormal. More commonly, the child seems to function poorly in one or more processes, with a learning problem the result. Some children learn better by listening to information, others by reading information. Most children will find their own best learning style. Some children with greater weaknesses in one area will require special help to get around their areas of difficulty and to maximize their strengths.

A child who is having learning problems in school, whether he has epilepsy or not, should receive a careful psychological and educational evaluation to identify his areas of strengths and weaknesses. Only then will the teachers be able to find the best way to help that child to learn. For some children this will mean extra help. For others it may require resource teachers with special training. For still others it may mean repeating a grade, being placed in a slower class, or being placed in a special education class. Each child and his problems are unique. The child and his problems must be individually assessed and a plan developed to meet that child's specific needs. All of these statements are true for the child with learning problems, *whether or not that child has epilepsy.* They are not different for the child with epilepsy, the problems are only more common.

## Attention Problems and Hyperactivity

In order to learn, you must pay attention to what is being taught. Teachers know that the attention span of young children is short. Therefore they teach in short blocks of time interspersed with activities such as marching around the room or recess. As the child gets older (as the nervous system and attention span mature), the child is able to sit and to concentrate or attend for increasingly long periods of time. Thus, a potential cause of a learning problem in the early years of school is that the child's nervous system is not yet sufficiently mature to allow the child to attend for long periods of time.

Another cause of attention problems could be that the child is not sufficiently bright to keep up with what is going on in the class and, therefore, is easily distracted. The other side of that coin is the very bright child who is bored by the slow pace of the class, her mind wandering to fill the time. A child who hasn't eaten and is hungry may also be less likely to pay attention. A child with insufficient sleep may have similar problems. There are many different reasons for a child's not paying attention in school.

A cause that has received much attention is a condition called "organic hyperactivity" or more recently "ADD," Attention Deficit Disorder. Although this condition is common, we know surprisingly little about its source. It may or may not be associated with physical hyperactivity. ADD is more common (or more easily recognized) in boys, where over-activity is a more common accompanying symptom and more likely to draw attention to the child. Attention Deficit Disorders are not uncommon in children during the early school years; they are perhaps even more common in children with epilepsy. They are also frequently associated with "immaturity" of the nervous system and with the learning disorders described above.

While its cause is unknown, we like to think of ADD as a "filtering" problem. Everyone is constantly bombarded by multiple different stimuli. As you are reading this chapter there may be children playing in the room, the TV may be playing, the clock ticking, and someone else talking. And yet you are able to filter all of these other stimuli out and concentrate, pay attention to what you are reading. We do not know exactly how this filtering takes place, but it seems to be partly a learned skill and partly a result of maturity of the nervous system. Infants and young children are easily distracted by the many stimuli around them; they have difficulty paying attention (except to TV). As they get older, they can attend better. Some children mature faster in this respect than others. Some have far more difficulty paying attention than others and are diagnosed as having Attention Deficit Disorders when the problem interferes with their work in school.

Some medications decrease a child's ability to pay attention, others appear to increase the child's ability to attend. Perhaps the actions of these drugs are on the "filter," either allowing more stimuli to reach consciousness and thus to be distracting, or increasing the filtering so the child is less aware of the distractions and can concentrate better.

Phenobarbital is known to increase the inattentiveness of some children and to cause hyperactivity as well. One of its actions may be to depress the "filter," allowing more distractions to reach conscious levels. Other drugs such as methylphenidate (Ritalin) and dextroamphetamine (Dexedrine) may act by improving the "filter" of inattentive (or hyperactive) children, allowing them to concentrate better. These drugs are often called stimulants because in older children and adults they seem to boost energy. Another medication, magnesium pemoline (Cylert), which does not have much effect on normal children or adults, but which is effective in children with ADD, may work in a similar manner.

*When a child with epilepsy is having difficulty focusing his attention, we need to ask if his anticonvulsant medication may be the cause. All anticonvulsants can cause both attention and learning problems. Phenobarbital seems to be the most frequent offender. Every parent of a child with epilepsy should be aware of his child's school performance and note if there is a change (for better or worse) when the child is started on medication, when the medication is changed to a new drug, OR when the dosage is increased.*

## Psychological and Social Problems

A child's performance at school is, to a large extent, determined by the child's feelings about himself. The child who thinks that he is dumb will frequently act and perform as if he is. He is unlikely to perform at his best level. The child who is depressed because of her seizures, because of his family's reaction to the seizures, or for other reasons is likely to do less well in school. Indeed, a drop in school performance may be one of the early signs of childhood depression.

But a child's school performance is also affected by what others think of him. Children, and even rats, tend to perform up to the levels of expectation. In a classic psychological experiment, researchers who were given rats to test, and who were told that they were studying "dumb rats," found that the rats did less well on testing than when they were studying "smart rats." This was true even when the "smart rats" and the "dumb rats" were brothers and sisters from the same litters with identical intelligence.

This can present a problem for the child with epilepsy and for that child's parents. If the child's teacher expects the child with epilepsy to have learning problems, then those problems are more likely to be found, whether they are present or not. On the other hand, a teacher who is aware that your child could have a learning problem is also more likely to identify the problem early and to be more sensitive to it. Therefore, telling the teacher about your child's epilepsy and about any concerns you may have about your child's learning could be an advantage to your child.

Make sure that the teacher understands about your child's type of seizures and that she makes you aware of any concerns she may have about your child and about any changes in your child's performance. These could be due to changes in medication or in the frequency or type of seizures. Mutual trust between you and your child's teacher and exchange of information and concerns can serve to benefit your child.

Here are some typical school problems we have seen:

**Mrs. Christiansen brought us a letter from Billy's teacher.**

**"We have enjoyed having Billy in our kindergarten this year. He is a charming, adorable little boy. However, he did so poorly on his reading readiness test that we all feel that he should spend another year in kindergarten. We would like you to come in for a meeting with us at your convenience."**

**"Doctor, should we tell her about Billy's epilepsy? He hasn't had a seizure since he started taking phenobarbital more than a year ago."**

The first thing we would recommend is that you and your husband meet with the teacher. Find out more about Billy's problems in school. Have there been other problems, or did he just do poorly on the reading readiness test? Is he immature in other ways in school? How does his ability to learn games and other things compare to his peers? Does the teacher think that this is just a problem of maturity which would be solved by repeating kindergarten, or are there other problems as well?

Teachers usually have a great deal of experience in identifying school problems, and the teacher's impressions can be of great help to you and to your physician in sorting out the problems and in finding the proper directions to proceed.

The second step would be to meet with us to get our advice about the teacher's impressions and suggestions. Do we all agree with the school? Is Billy one of the younger children in the class who could benefit from another year? Is he immature in other social ways? Does he act more like a five-year-old than the usual six-year-old who is starting first grade? Is he intellectually slower than normal? Is he a child with a specific learning problem? We often cannot answer these last two questions without psychological testing.

Does every child who is like Billy need testing? We would say no, but whether a child does or does not need testing will depend on the opinion of the teacher and on our assessment. We are often asked to answer the question, "Is this neurological?" Our answer is always, "Yes. Learning problems are always neurological." Learning resides in the brain, not in the foot or heart. If a child isn't learning, it's because he can't or doesn't use his brain as expected. This does NOT mean that Billy has a neurological problem or that he needs to see a neurologist. It means that all of us (including the teacher) need to assess the situation carefully and find the best educational strategy to manage the problem.

Those are the suggestions we would give to *any* parents who received that note from their child's teacher. The only thing different about Billy is that he has seizures and is on phenobarbital. Yes, you should tell the teacher about Billy's seizures. You might also ask her if she has seen any "daydreaming" or other evidence that he may have been having subtle seizures in school. We would also be concerned about the possible role of the phenobarbital. We would recommend checking the blood level of phenobarbital to see if it is too high and interfering with Billy's learning. We would probably recommend changing to another anticonvulsant (if Billy needed to continue medication) to see if his performance improved. *There is no way to be absolutely certain that the medication is not interfering with learning and behavior except to take the child off of that medicine and, if necessary, change to another medicine.*

**"This was the third time this fall that the teacher has called us in for a meeting. She says that Joshua is disruptive to the class. He bites, fights, and won't sit still. His reading is terrible, and I'm afraid that he is going to be expelled. What should we do? Can they expel someone from the second grade? I think that the real problem is that the teacher is afraid that he'll have a seizure in class and really just wants him out."**

We would begin to analyze this problem by asking the parents to tell us more about Joshua. What sort of a child is he? Is he having these types of behavior problems at home? Are they new? When did they first start? Was he having similar problems in the first grade last year? Was there anything particular which might have caused them? What was the relationship of the onset of these problems to the onset of his seizures and to the initiation of his anticonvulsant medication?

Behavioral problems such as biting, fighting, and other disruptive behavior can come from many different sources. Any of the anticonvulsant medications can cause behavioral changes such as this. If the change began shortly after the start of a new anticonvulsant, then perhaps a different medication should be tried. However, behavioral changes rarely occur weeks or months after the child has been on the same medicine, unless there has been a change in the dose. New behavior problems can be caused by psychological disturbances initiated by problems at home or in school; they could be caused by the teacher's behavior towards the child and the child's reaction to his teacher's behavior. Does Joshua know about his seizures? Is he afraid or embarrassed by them? Perhaps a careful explanation of the seizures would alleviate some of his fears, and this might allow him to be less aggressive in school.

Discussing the problems and concerns with the teacher (or the principal) and with your physician can help you to sort through these different causes. Whatever the cause, the recent change in Josh's behavior certainly is reason for concern and investigation. It is a common symptom of problems that require solutions. It could be Joshua's psychological way of asking for help.

**"Martha's grades are terrible. She was a solid 'B' student until her seizure, and since then she doesn't even finish her homework. Her last report card was 'C's and 'D's, and she now says that she wants to drop out of school and get a job. Could this be due to her medicine?"**

In Martha's case, as in Joshua's, there are many potential sources for her problems. Puberty, boys, home problems, changes in school, depression, concern and embarrassment over her seizures could all affect school work and should be explored in talking with Martha. We would check the blood level and lower it if it was high. If not, we would strongly consider changing to another medicine. While phenobarbital and phenytoin are the medications that most frequently affect learning, such effects can follow use of *any* of the medications. Even as we were lowering or changing the medicine, we would explore with Martha what she knows about seizures and her reaction to them. We would want to know how seizures have changed her lifestyle and her sense of self-esteem. We would ask about symptoms of depression and try to help her cope better with her epilepsy, whether or not this was the cause of her school problems.

**"Circe's teacher called us this week because she is daydreaming in class. We had told her to watch for seizures in the beginning of the year, and now she thinks that Circe is having absence seizures again. Should we increase her medicine?"**

Circe could be having more absence seizures. Perhaps this alert teacher has identified the problem early. Have you seen any at home? Is Circe aware of missing things? Is it possible that the teacher is just watching too closely and misinterpreting things? Perhaps we should first check the blood level to be certain that she is taking the medication and taking enough. Perhaps we should see Circe and hyperventilate her to see if we can produce one of her spells. If we can't be sure in the office, we might want to have another EEG to see if she is still having electrical spells. In this way we can sort out if Circe has a problem and the best approach to correcting it.

*Learning problems are more common in children who have epilepsy. Early identification of a problem, if it exists, can lead to strategies for compensation and a far more successful school learning experience. However, learning problems can also be secondary to the medication, to psychological stress, and to the school's and the teacher's reaction to the child and to epilepsy. Changes in school performance are best identified by the teacher, who, together with your physician, can also be your and your child's best ally in finding the cause and the best approach to a solution.*

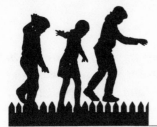

# 20. Common Sense: Sports and Epilepsy

Participation in sports is an important part of the process of growing up. There are, of course, marked variations in individuals' athletic ability, in their stage of development, in their coordination, and in their interest in sports. Whether group play during recess, team sports like Little League, soccer, and football, or individual sports like swimming, tennis, and riding, sports are important to a child's personal and social development. They offer an opportunity to participate with others, to share, to learn teamwork and self-discipline, skills important to the development of personality, self-esteem, confidence, and character. *No one should be deprived of those opportunities.*

Participation in organizations, such as Scouts, clubs, church groups, and so on, can also be important to the development of self-esteem and character. Children with epilepsy are less likely to be excluded from these organizations than they are from sports.

In our paternalistic approach to children, and particularly our paternalistic approach to children with problems or potential problems, we often restrict the child from opportunities for participation. Sports are one notable area for such restrictions. There is little reason for these restrictions. We should not paternalistically superimpose handicap on disability. Risk-benefit analysis and decision-making are the principles that should govern decisions about a child's participation in sports.

*No blanket statement about sports participation for persons with epilepsy is possible. Decisions about participation must be based on an individual's circumstances, the type of seizure, and his or her degree of seizure control. The decision must, further, be based on risks of the particular sport and the accommodations that can feasibly be made for that individual.*

*The rules governing participation of children with epilepsy in sports should, in other words, be based on common sense! Each decision should be individualized.*

**"My son loves to play contact sports. He was a football player, on the freshman wrestling team, and played lacrosse. Now that he has had a seizure, the coach won't let him participate. He is crestfallen. What should we do?"**

If your son has had a single generalized tonic-clonic seizure, and your physician has found no reason for the seizure, there is probably no reason why he should not resume his sports. If he had a complex partial seizure, then this may have been the first recognized seizure; his physician has probably started medication. For a time, it might be wise to allow him to practice with the team, but to refrain from game situations where a momentary lapse of attention might cause injury. When medication has controlled the seizures without side effects, then he can resume playing.

**"Does he need to wear a special helmet to protect his head when he's playing?"**

The brain of someone with epilepsy usually is no more sensitive or susceptible to injury than that of anyone else. In contact sports where headgear is required, that headgear should be sufficient for the child with epilepsy. Trauma to the head, which occurs in all of these sports, is unlikely to precipitate a seizure.

**"The doctor had him hyperventilate in the office. It didn't cause a seizure, but could running hard and being out of breath cause a seizure while he is playing?"**

No. Hyperventilation during exercise is balanced by changes in body chemistry and cannot produce a seizure. We took care of one young woman who was so sensitive to hyperventilation that with only a few deep breaths she would experience seizures we could show our medical students every time she came to clinic for her check-up. Yet she was a long-distance bicycle rider and never had a seizure while riding.

*"Jennifer wants to go on the Outward Bound trip this summer. We still haven't been able to get complete control of her absence seizures. They aren't often, but suppose one occurred while she was on one of those rope swings?"*

If a spell occurred while she was on a rope, she could fall and hurt herself. On the other hand, anyone in the group who fell from the rope could injure himself, so the group leader should be quite careful. Perhaps you and Jennifer should talk with the leader. Maybe she could join the trip but avoid doing some of the most dangerous things. The independence taught by the trip and the benefits of being part of the group might be good for her and might also help her to realize that everyone has some limitations, at times. If her seizures were under control, her risks of injury would be little greater than those of others on the trip, and she could participate fully.

*"Edith is eight and wants to go to one of those sports camps where they do gymnastics, work on the bars and the trampolines. Should I let her go?"*

Everyone who exercises on a trampoline should be carefully supervised. If Edith is having frequent seizures, whether they are big seizures or staring spells, it's preferable that she not fall great distances. So she probably should not work on a high bar—or climb trees, either. However, if her seizures are controlled, if she continues to take her medicine, then her chances of injury are not much greater than the other children's. All child gymnasts need a soft place to land. It does not have to be softer for children with epilepsy. There should, of course, be mats and appropriate protection, both for any child who makes a mistake and for the child who might have a seizure.

*"Bobbie wants to go out for cheerleading. They do all sorts of acrobatic stunts. What do you think?"*

Surprisingly, cheerleading, which we think of as a girls' sport, probably presents the greatest risk of injury of any high school sport. In the past there were no coaches, no training, no rules—and hard gym floors. The least coordinated individual used to be placed on the top of the pyramid! That's dumb, for the individual with epilepsy and for the one without. With adequate coaching and training, cheerleading should be no more risky for someone with controlled epilepsy than for the child who hasn't had seizures.

***"Can David play soccer? Will hitting the ball with his head hurt him or cause a seizure?"***

There is no evidence that hitting the soccer ball with his head will injure the brain or precipitate seizures.

***"What about water sports—swimming, rowing, and sailing?"***

Water sports are all potentially dangerous sports since even adults can drown. When anyone swims or dives there should always be adequate supervision. These sports present a minimally greater risk for the child with epilepsy, proportional to the frequency and the type of seizures. When these sports are competitive, the risk is probably decreased, since the competitors are being closely observed. In boating, anyone can capsize, tumble into the water, or be knocked unconscious and into the water by the boom. All sailors should wear life jackets. Then they will be protected, even if they have seizures.

The same premise applies to all children. If a child could be injured in a sport, then there should be adequate protection to prevent or minimize an injury and adequate supervision to treat the injury if an accident occurs. For the child with seizures, the same is true. If a child has just started having seizures or has just started on new medication, then more supervision should be provided, and perhaps even a bit of overprotection until the seizures are controlled or the degree of seizure control is ascertained. When the child has fewer seizures, or no seizures at all, he doesn't need extra protection.

***"My daughter is a competitive swimmer. She feels that her anticonvulsant medication slows her down and tends to skip it on the days before her meets. I'm afraid that she will have a seizure. What should I tell her?"***

You should tell her that the medication is far less likely than a seizure to interfere with her performance. You should make a contract with her that if she is mature enough to take training and swimming seriously, then she is also mature enough to manage her seizures and to take her medication reliably. If she feels that the medications are slowing her down, she should discuss this with her doctor. Perhaps he can lower the dose. But your daughter should not do this on her own. Perhaps the medication could even be discontinued if she has been seizure-free for a sufficient period of time.

*"We've just moved to a new town, and Todd hasn't had a seizure in almost a year. Should he tell his coach that he has epilepsy?"*

Yes. That is the only way the coach can provide adequate supervision and be prepared if another seizure occurs. If the coach acts in a paternalistic way, then you may have a battle to fight. It is important that you and your child be honest with the coach, just as you expect him to be honest with you.

*"Would you let an adolescent with epilepsy participate in a marathon or in one of those triathalons? Does the stress of these increase the chance of seizures?"*

In general, stress of this sort does not increase the chance of a seizure. The training for the event might provide a very good test. We would allow him to try. If the training seemed to increase the frequency of seizures, he should probably not compete. If he's had seizures before, he might be distressed if he had another one, but it would probably be less distressing than if he hasn't even been allowed to try.

*"It sounds as if you would allow a child with epilepsy to do almost anything that they're capable of. Is that correct?"*

Yes. We think a little common sense goes a long way. The most common problems for children with epilepsy are the paternalism of the physician and of society and overprotection by families. Sports are an excellent way for your child to develop skills and self-confidence. These skills will be useful in adult life, whether or not the seizures are cured or controlled. Children with epilepsy have enough problems without being made to feel different because of the overprotectiveness of others who fear another seizure.

We are far more permissive than many physicians. You or your doctor may put more restrictions on what your child can do, with or without epilepsy. The risks of participation in a particular sport will vary with your child and his seizures. The benefits of a particular sport also vary with the child. Participation in a sport like football may or may not be very important to your child. You and your child will have to weigh both the risks and the benefits of participation. Your physician may be a good advisor.

*Sports, particularly competitive sports, are about participation, about being a member of a team. They're about trying to be the best at something. They're about self-esteem. Sports seem to be good for most children; perhaps they are even more important for the child with epilepsy.*

# 21. Driving and Epilepsy

Driving is risky business for everyone. The magnitude of the risk of driving is determined by the driver's age, sex, and use of drugs and alcohol. Health problems such as diabetes, stroke, heart disease, and prior health-related incidents like head trauma and infections of the nervous system can also be risk factors. Epilepsy is only one health-related condition that carries a risk factor for driving.

Driving is considered a privilege, and, therefore, people are licensed to drive. In granting that privilege, society theoretically weighs the risks to the public of granting the license against the benefits to the individual of being able to drive. In the U.S. a state grants or withdraws the privilege. What are the risks to society of someone driving who has epilepsy? What benefits does an individual lose when a license is not granted?

Because seizures are transient alterations of consciousness or of motor or sensory function, caused by electrical discharges from the brain, it is obvious that some of these alterations, in particular, of consciousness, can lead to a motor vehicle accident if they occur while the person is driving. Not all seizures do involve loss of consciousness. Some are purely sensory. Some may be purely focal motor. Neither of these may interfere with control of the car. Some persons experience an aura (warning) before a seizure, allowing the driver to pull off the road. Some seizures occur only during sleep. To be reasonable and sensible,

Information in this section was heavily drawn from the excellent review by A. Krumholtz, R. S. Fisher, R. P. Lesser, and A. Hauser, "Driving and Epilepsy: A Review and Reappraisal." *JAMA*. In press.

licensing procedures should be guided by the type of seizure the individual has.

It is estimated that while one in ten persons has a single seizure at *some time* during a lifetime, only a small proportion of these will have a second seizure, and even if an individual did have a second seizure, it would be unlikely to occur during the tiny fraction of his life that is spent driving. For most individuals who do experience a second seizure (epilepsy), seizures are controlled by medication; as long as the individual takes his medication the risk of further recurrence remains low. Thus, there is even more reason to individualize rules about driving.

The chances of having a recurrence while driving will obviously be determined in part by the amount of time the person spends at the wheel. That risk is also affected by sleeplessness, by use of other medications, and by many unknown factors.

*Thus, it is impossible to make any blanket statements about* ALL *people with epilepsy and equally impossible to make blanket statements about the chance of a recurrence while a person with epilepsy is driving. The risks of recurrence and the risks of driving must be assessed individually.*

With these caveats, one study found that only one accident in 10,000 was due to a seizure while driving; six were due to natural death at the wheel. Alcohol was responsible for 2,500 of the 10,000 accidents studied. Some studies do suggest that the traffic accident rate may be higher for those with epilepsy, but also that women *with* epilepsy have a lower accident rate than men *without* epilepsy. The rate of accidents for persons with epilepsy is no different from the rate for those with cardiovascular disease or diabetes. It has been estimated that in only one in five accidents involving a person with epilepsy is the accident the result of a seizure, and that those accidents, in fact, tend to be less severe, to involve only a driver's vehicle, and to occur in less populated areas. Therefore, even when epilepsy might contribute to an accident, that accident appears to present, in general, less risk to others.

The risks and consequences of not being allowed to drive are also quite individual, depending on where the individual lives, the availability of alternative transportation, the need to drive to get to college or a job, and the social consequences of the resulting isolation. In this country, for example, driving is often an economic and social necessity.

Although at one time few people with epilepsy were permitted to drive at all, in recent years there has been an increasing tendency to liberalize the restrictions and to individualize the limitations on driving. Laws regarding restrictions vary state by state in the U.S. and country by country. Some states have no restrictions, provided the physician gives permission to drive; in others a person with epilepsy must have been free of seizures for three months to one year before driving. Most states have medical panels and appeals processes to review applications, but these panels often do not include neurologists or others with knowledge and experience with epilepsy.

Reporting requirements for seizures are confusing and differ from state to state. Very few states require the physician to report the name of an individual who has had seizures; however, when a physician feels that an individual presents a "substantial risk to others" because the individual is driving against medical advice, reporting may be necessary. Physicians whose patients have continued seizures should warn them of the risks involved with continued driving and document this warning in writing.

Persons with epilepsy should be aware of and obey the local regulations affecting their driving. Failure to follow regulations may result in accidents. Accidents occurring when the driver's epilepsy is unreported, even if unrelated to a seizure, can result in problems with insurance coverage. Check with your physician and your motor vehicle administration for applicable regulations. The most common regulation is that the individual be seizure-free for a designated period of time before driving. All of these time periods are arbitrary. Studies show that a person who is seizure-free for three months has an 85 percent chance of remaining seizure-free the next year. Based on these studies we recommend that the regulations be changed to a three-month waiting period.

Seizures that are a result of changes in medication at a physician's direction should not necessarily limit driving privileges. If you had a seizure while your physician was decreasing your medicine, resumption of your previous dosage should re-establish seizure control and you should be able to continue to drive.

Individuals who have epilepsy controlled with medication and whose physicians are now recommending discontinuing medication pose special dilemmas for both the physician and the driver. Optimally, we would like to help patients be free of medication if possible. While in an ideal patient the risk of recurrent seizures is small, if they recur it is most likely to happen in the first three to six months after stopping medication. Most physicians recommend that the patient should *not* drive during that period of increased risk. If driving is absolutely essential, then risks should be minimized by limiting the amount of time behind the wheel. Driving while tired or for long distances should be avoided during this period.

Clearly there is need for better information on the risks of driving with epilepsy. Such information should assess the risks of recurrence of seizures and factors which are predictive of such a recurrence, as well as the risks and hazards of accidents and of injuries to others. These risks should be placed in the perspective of other health-related disabilities. The driving risks represented by persons who use drugs and alcohol far outweigh the risks associated with epilepsy. These factors should be considered by the regulating agency when deciding whose driving should be restricted and for how long. The availability of restricted licenses that might permit an individual to drive to work or to school or only under certain restricted circumstances might balance the public's risk of allowing some people with epilepsy to drive against the high cost of restricting the privilege.

*Above all, decisions about driving need to be based on individual needs and capacities.*

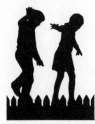

# 22. Marriage, Pregnancy, and Children

Parents rightfully wonder and worry about their child's future. Marriage and grandchildren are a part of that future. Not so long ago, marriage of persons with epilepsy was prohibited by law in many states. The eugenics movement, relying on a U.S. Supreme Court decision and on the principle that "one generation of imbeciles is enough," was able to implement these laws. Fortunately, the erroneous rationale behind these laws was disproved and the laws abolished. Ironically, we are only now beginning to gain significant information about the genetics of the epilepsies. Many misconceptions and misbeliefs still abound, for example, about the effects of pregnancy on epilepsy and about the effects of epilepsy and its treatment on a fetus. Physicians themselves often give outdated answers to these questions.

## Marriage and Parenthood

### "Can I get married?"

Of course! If you are competent to be a spouse, however that competence is defined, there is no reason why a person with epilepsy should not get married.

### "Can I have children?"

Yes. Most women with epilepsy can bear children.

*"Can a person with epilepsy be a competent parent?"*

The answer is clearly, "Yes!" Most people who have epilepsy are extremely competent parents, just as are most people without. Some are incompetent parents, just as are some without epilepsy. Individuals with epilepsy have personal strengths and weaknesses just as others do. You will have to ask yourself and your partner whether you as individuals have the ability, maturity, and judgment to be good parents. That is for you to decide, but a "no" decision should not be based simply on the fact that you have epilepsy.

*"Can someone who still has seizures be a good parent?"*

Absolutely, although the problems of being a parent with ongoing seizures may be more difficult. If your seizures are frequent and result in sudden loss of consciousness, you might drop or injure your child during a seizure. You may have to make arrangements for special help in the home or special arrangements for child care outside the home. But even so, you can be a good parent.

## Risks of Pregnancy and of Anticonvulsant Drugs

Although pregnancy might affect your seizures, your risks during pregnancy are little different from the risks other women face. If you have questions about conditions that might have caused your epilepsy or about the effect of pregnancy on other health problems, you should check with your physician *before* you decide to become pregnant.

Your seizures may change during pregnancy. Therefore, your obstetrician needs to know about your epilepsy and your neurologist about your pregnancy. In about one-third of pregnant women, seizures get worse, in one-third they improve, and in one-third they are unchanged. Since we cannot predict which group you will fall into, your pregnancy should be monitored carefully. Ideally you should be on the lowest amount of a drug, and on a single drug only, to control your seizures. This drug, and its level, should, if possible, be determined before you become pregnant. Anticonvulsants should not be changed during your pregnancy unless such a change is needed for seizure control or because of toxicity.

Since blood levels change as your body chemistry itself changes during the pregnancy, blood levels of your medications should be monitored. We generally recommend that these levels should be measured early in the pregnancy, then followed every month in the middle third of your pregnancy and every several weeks in the last trimester.

There are three principal reasons why seizures increase during pregnancy in almost one of three women with epilepsy. The first is that pregnant women are naturally fearful that taking drugs may affect the fetus and, therefore, may fail to take anticonvulsant medication according to schedule. A second reason is lack of sleep during pregnancy. A third cause of seizures during pregnancy is changes in the body's metabolism of drugs. Although such changes can cause blood levels to rise and thus cause toxicity, blood levels can also decline, leading to seizures. Your physician should closely follow your blood levels and provide appropriate adjustments.

Although there is little evidence that brief seizures injure the fetus, a prolonged seizure might affect your fetus and any seizures might cause injury to you. Therefore, we strongly urge that pregnant women with epilepsy who need medication for seizure control continue to take the drug that has been controlling their seizures.

### *"Are there risks to my baby when I am taking anticonvulsant drugs?"*

Yes, there are risks of anticonvulsant drugs to the baby. Those risks vary with the drug and are usually small.

*No pregnant woman should be on anticonvulsant medication if it is not needed.*

Every pregnancy with epilepsy or without carries some risk of having an abnormal baby. Approximately 2 percent of all children will be born with some developmental abnormality. When a woman either has, or has previously had, epilepsy but is not taking medication during the pregnancy, the risk of a child with an abnormality is 4 to 5 percent (almost twice as high as the baseline 2 percent). Thus, this woman has a 95 percent chance of having a normal infant. Some studies suggest that this risk is not increased by taking anticonvulsants. Other studies say that the risk of abnormality in such a case could be as high as 7 to 17 percent. Even if we accept the highest estimate as correct, the chance of having a normal child is still 80 to 90 percent. The chances of having an abnormal child are also increased when the father has epilepsy, although the risks are less high.

*Each medicine may pose different risks to the fetus, some more serious than others, and some may cause problems more frequently.*

Abnormalities vary with the anticonvulsant and may be severe—

such as spina bifida, congenital heart disease, or cleft palate—or minor abnormalities in appearance as in the length of the fingernails.

*Trimethadione (Tridione) and paramethadione (Paradione).* These drugs should never be used during pregnancy because of the very high incidence of serious malformations in babies of mothers taking them.

*Phenytoin (Dilantin).* This drug is believed by most people to carry an increased risk of cleft lip and palate, as well as of congenital heart disease. The risk of these problems is about 5 percent. Since these malformations occur during the first weeks of pregnancy, they cannot be prevented by stopping the drug after you realize you are pregnant. It is alleged that there is an increase in risk of "fetal hydantoin syndrome" when the mother has been taking phenytoin. In this syndrome, the infant has short distal fingers and toes, small fingernails, is of slightly short stature, and has a small head. Whether such children are intellectually disabled or not remains a matter of debate. Some people feel that the risk of this syndrome is perhaps 20 to 30 percent. Others feel that the significance of these minor abnormalities is greatly overstated. Similar features may be found in children of a mother with epilepsy who has taken phenobarbital (the fetal barbiturate syndrome) and one who has not been on medication at all.

Fetal hydantoin syndrome may be caused by the way certain women metabolize the drug. If you have a baby who has had the syndrome your chances of having another affected child may be very high if you continue taking phenytoin (Dilantin) during your second pregnancy.

*Phenobarbital.* This drug causes exactly the same complications as phenytoin—the cleft and heart problems and the "fetal barbiturate syndrome"—but the chances of each occurring appears to be slightly less than with phenytoin.

*Valproic Acid (Depakene, Depakote).* This drug has been found to increase the risk of malformations, particularly of spinal cord problems (spina bifida), to a rate of 1 to 2 percent. Women taking valproic acid should discuss risks with their physicians before becoming pregnant because it may be possible to substitute another medication. Women who become pregnant while on this drug should ask their physicians about a special blood test that might detect spina bifida early in the pregnancy.

*Carbamazepine (Tegretol).* This drug has been less well studied than other anticonvulsants. Although it, too, has been associated with problems for the fetus, it appears to be one of the safer anticonvulsants.

*A woman who no longer needs medication should have it discon-
tinued before she becomes pregnant. This should be done under a
physician's supervision. For the woman in whom the need for continued medication is unclear, decision-making can be complex.*

It is likely that all medications in pregnancy will pose some minimal
risk to the fetus. Virtually all anticonvulsants may affect the metabolism of vitamin K in the newborn and may lead to bleeding. Therefore,
the mother should receive vitamin K during the last week of pregnancy,
or the infant should receive it immediately after birth.

❏ **Barbara was thirty-one and desperately wanted to have a child. She had
recently been placed on phenytoin because of a single seizure. She had a
dilemma. Should she get pregnant with the risks of medication to the fetus or
should she stop the medication with the risks of a seizure to herself and the
fetus? Although she realized that the risks of phenytoin (Dilantin) to her baby
were small, she could not accept the guilt of potentially causing a problem. She
was also fearful of having a seizure while she was pregnant and of possibly
injuring the baby. She was much less concerned about the potential effects of a
seizure on her own active life.**

**We suggested a way out of her dilemma. Since she had only had a single
seizure, the chances of her having another seizure were approximately 30 percent. If her medication was slowly discontinued, she could wait three to six
months and see if another seizure occurred. After that time the risk of recurrence would be even smaller and she could become pregnant with greater
security. If she had another seizure, then she would know that she needed an
anticonvulsant medication and might try one with less potential risk to the
fetus.**

*If you become pregnant while you are on anticonvulsants, you
should be reassured that at least 80 to 90 percent of the babies will be
normal. Pregnancy is not a good time to stop taking the medication or
to switch to another drug, unless it is necessary for your seizure control.*

## Breastfeeding and Birth Control

*"Can I breastfeed my baby?"*

Yes. While all of the anticonvulsants are found in breast milk, they are usually in such low concentrations that they do not affect the baby. However, if you are taking phenobarbital or phenytoin and the baby becomes too sleepy, then the baby's blood level should be checked. If the level is too high, breastfeeding might be stopped for a few days.

*"What about birth control?"*

Anticonvulsants increase the metabolism of birth control steroids and make them less effective. Therefore, if you are using birth control pills, particularly the "mini-pill," and are taking anticonvulsants, you might have a higher chance of becoming pregnant. You should discuss this with your physician.

## "Will My Child Be Normal?"

*"Since I have seizures, are there any risks of my child developing epilepsy?"*

Yes, there is a small risk of your children developing epilepsy. The risk of epilepsy in the child whose mother or father has epilepsy is about twice as great as when neither of the parents has epilepsy but still relatively small. The risk of anybody's child having epilepsy is 1 to 2 percent. Because you have epilepsy, your child has a 3 to 4 percent chance of having epilepsy.

*"If I have a child will he or she be normal?"*

No one can give you a warranty on your child. Some abnormalities are not detectable even by our most sophisticated prenatal and intra-uterine screening. Some major problems are acquired at birth or are a consequence of later infection or trauma. Some genetic diseases cause epilepsy. Some risks are associated with anticonvulsants. There are some risks if you have previously had epilepsy.

*If you are unwilling to take any risk, then you should probably not have a child. If you are willing to take a small risk, then you, as well as most people with epilepsy, can have healthy and normal children.*

## Other Genetic Issues

Some people ask us about the risks for their child if other family members have epilepsy. Some parents who do not have epilepsy themselves ask about risks for subsequent children when one of their children has had seizures. The answers to these questions require more detailed explanation.

Epilepsy may be a manifestation of some other disease. Some metabolic diseases, such as the aminoacidurias like phenylketonuria (PKU), and degenerative diseases, like Tay-Sachs and metachromatic leukodystrophy, may cause seizures. If one of your children has such a metabolic disease, the risk of a subsequent child's having it is one in four. That other child is also likely to have seizures. If your brother or sister had the condition and you did not, you might carry the gene. If you do, and if you were unlucky enough to marry someone else who also had the same abnormal gene, then the chance of your child's being affected could be as high as one in four. If you do not carry the abnormal gene, your chances of having an affected child are zero.

In a few diseases such as tuberous sclerosis or neurofibromatosis, the recurrence rate may be as high as one in two. If you, as the parent, had tuberous sclerosis, for example, half of your children could also have the disease and may have seizures.

If one of your children has idiopathic seizures, seizures for which the cause cannot be identified, the chances of other children also having seizures is twice as high as in the general population. Thus, they would have a 3 to 4 percent chance of having epilepsy. If one of your children has a febrile seizure, or a seizure after head trauma, the chances of brothers and sisters having similar seizures are also twice as high as the general population.

*In summary, there is a genetic tendency to inheriting epilepsy, but the risk is small both for the child of a person who has epilepsy and for her brothers and sisters.*

# 23. Support Services:
## The Epilepsy Foundation of America and Its Affiliates

When parents face a diagnosis of epilepsy, in addition to the shock and grief most also suffer from the same ignorance and misunderstandings that afflict the general public. You need information. You need someone or some group to talk to. You need support. Where do you turn? Whom do you go to who has had a child with epilepsy and who can help you to understand? What is the best approach to coping?

Your doctor and his staff will be a major source of information and support. Further outside support can be obtained from the Epilepsy Foundation of America.

The Epilepsy Foundation of America (EFA) is the national organization that represents people with epilepsy. Together with its independent local affiliates scattered across the country, EFA is the best repository of information about epilepsy and about treatment and solutions to the everyday problems of living with epilepsy. This information is available free by calling either your local affiliate (usually listed in the phone book) or the Epilepsy Foundation's national office on a toll free line, 1-800-EFA-1000 (in Maryland, call 301-459-3700).

EFA is far more than an information and referral service. It is a major national organization that advocates legislation and provides services, education, and resources to you and your child.

"That's all very nice," you say, "but I don't need advocacy, I need help and information." You may feel all you need is help right now, but over the longer term, you and your child and all other people with epilepsy need advocacy, too. The Epilepsy Foundation of America provides *both* help and advocacy.

*Only by working together can persons with epilepsy and their families learn about the causes of epilepsy, improve treatment of the condition, and hope to find a cure. Together, all families touched by epilepsy can help each person with this disorder achieve full potential. Only together can we overcome the misunderstandings that handicap us all.*

Did you know that it was EFA that pushed Congress to establish a National Commission on the Epilepsies in 1975? This commission spent several years reviewing the problems faced by people with epilepsy, their families, and communities. It made specific recommendations for action nationwide, some of which are detailed below:

• The Commission highlighted the need for new medications to control seizures. Some of these medications were already available in Europe, but not in the United States.
• The Commission emphasized how little we knew about the condition and pressed for additional research in needed areas and more funding to support it.
• The Commission recommended the establishment of a national information center to provide up-to-date information about epilepsy. The Epilepsy Foundation has created such a center.
• It uncovered gaps in the laws protecting children and adults with epilepsy and recommended changes. This enabled children with epilepsy to benefit from Public Law 94–142, the Education for All Handicapped Children Act, which assures appropriate education in the least restrictive environment for every child. Earlier, many children with seizures were forced to receive their education, if any, at home because schools were afraid that seizures would occur on their premises.
• The Commission recommended that persons with epilepsy receive the benefits of vocational training already being offered to other disabled individuals.

Many other suggestions were embodied in the Commission's multivolume report, but the Commission's own role was to survey the present situation and develop a national plan of action. It was not empowered to make necessary changes.

The Epilepsy Foundation of America has assumed responsibility for overseeing the Commission's recommendations, for actively lobbying Congress and governmental agencies to implement these recommendations, and for implementing many of the Commission's recommendations itself.

Among the changes EFA has helped to bring about are these:

• Inclusion of children with epilepsy in education legislation benefiting the handicapped. Legislation such as PL 94–142, the Education For All Handicapped Act, prevents discrimination in the schools and ensures equal educational opportunities for all children. More recent bills (PL 99–148) mandate early educational opportunities for all handicapped children.
• Inclusion of people with epilepsy in vocational education and rehabilitation programs. The Epilepsy Foundation designed and has developed model job training programs, funded by the U.S. Department of Labor. These programs have consistently demonstrated that most individuals with epilepsy can benefit from job training and from acquiring job-seeking skills and can become gainfully employed as excellent workers.

More recently, the EFA has turned some of its attention to those even more handicapped with epilepsy to find ways to help them to become employable.

Perhaps the most important role for the national organization has been public education. It is helping to overcome the biases and prejudices about epilepsy. Through messages on national television and radio, EFA has shown both that normal people can and do have epilepsy and that people with epilepsy can be normal. Through nationally-televised programs, EFA has helped to educate the public and physicians about epilepsy and its proper management. Through literature and films directed to doctors, nurses, employers, schools, camp directors, and even to baby-sitters, the organization has reduced the mythology and prejudice and raised the level of knowledge and of understanding about epilepsy, and of the capabilities of children and adults with epilepsy.

The Foundation has developed a national Information and Referral Service to respond to your toll-free calls and answer your questions. EFA also will provide pamphlets and brochures that have been developed for parents, patients, school teachers, nurses, and other people involved with individuals who have epilepsy. It has established a National Epilepsy Library, a computerized comprehensive database of the various aspects of epilepsy. Physicians and other professionals can access the latest developments in the field of epilepsy by contacting the library (1-800-EFA-4050). The Foundation publishes a national newspaper, *The Spokesman,* distributed monthly to its membership, with up-to-date information about national and local progress in research and in services. It also provides a forum for parents and people with epilepsy to reach each other.

One problem that must be faced in informing other people about children with epilepsy is that there are really two different populations. One population of persons with epilepsy is perfectly normal; they generally have their seizures under control with medication or have recovered from epilepsy. For these people, the message must be that epilepsy is not a handicap, and there should be no discrimination. For the smaller population, those who continue to have seizures and those who have additional handicaps, the message must be different. These individuals clearly need help. They need research to find new medications and new approaches to control their seizures. They may need special programs in schools and in the workplace. They need parent- and family-support services. EFA's message is mindful of its dual role.

The Epilepsy Foundation of America is deeply committed to research to improve understanding of the mechanisms that underlie epilepsy and to find new approaches and medications for controlling seizures. Both through its close working relationships with the Epilepsy Branch of the National Institutes of Health, the principal NIH organization that sponsors research in epilepsy, and through its own fundraising efforts, the Foundation stimulates epilepsy research and supports promising young investigators.

Local affiliates of the Epilepsy Foundation of America exist in almost every state. While these affiliates vary in size and capabilities, each attempts to provide information, referral, and support services to people in their community with epilepsy and to their families. Some local affiliates have programs for teaching job-seeking skills, for job training, and other employment services. Some have self-help and support groups for parents whose children have epilepsy and for persons with epilepsy, including adolescents and children. Such groups can provide you or your child with the peers who can supply information and answer your questions.

Local affiliates have been creative in many special areas that can benefit you and your child. Some of their projects have included:

- Camps for children with epilepsy;
- Provision of trained speakers to present age-appropriate slide or film presentations about epilepsy in the schools;
- Special public school programs to provide guidance and placement;
- After-school programs and summer programs to provide work experience and training for success;
- Residential living programs for young adults who need training for independence. These programs provide varying levels of supervision and training to provide the skills necessary for self-support: for example, to use public transportation, to shop and cook, and to hold a job.

*You should join your local epilepsy association if you or your child need help; you or your child may be able to offer help to others who need it. You should also join the national organization, the Epilepsy Foundation of America, not only because of the effective job it is doing on a national level, but because individuals touched by epilepsy, those with the condition and their families, need to band together to make a better life for everyone with this condition.*

## Additional Readings and References

There are no references in this book. This is not an oversight. The information about epilepsy is changing and evolving. Most of it is not readily available to parents or in the local library.

The Epilepsy Foundation of America, through its national library, is the most current source of information. This information is available to you free of charge by writing to EFA or by calling their toll free number, 1-800-EFA-1000.

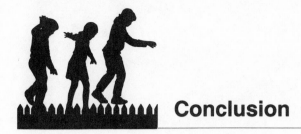

# Conclusion

We're not sure why you have read this book. Perhaps it was because you were shocked, upset, disheartened because your child has had a seizure or because she has been diagnosed as having epilepsy. Maybe you simply wanted to know more about seizures, their treatment, and their consequences. Whatever the reason, we hope that now you realize that epilepsy is not just a medical problem, but affects many other aspects of your child's life and of your life. We hope that now, more familiar with what epilepsy is and what epilepsy is not, you will raise your child in a far more optimistic and accepting fashion.

We wish you well. We hope that your child grows up without handicap, or with as little handicap as possible. We hope that you will learn to accept your child for whatever he or she may be and that you will help her fulfill her genuine potential and not impose handicaps. We hope that you have sensed our own personal involvement with each of our patients and that as you have read the stories of these children, you have sensed how each of these children has affected us, too. We have learned from each of them, and we hope that you will have learned as well. We hope that you and your child will find your own ways of coping.

Acceptance of seizures and their uncertainties, or of associated handicapping conditions, does not come easily and it does not mean resignation. Optimism may, at times, be hard to discover, but it is essential. We strongly believe that our optimistic approach is realistic. After all, most epilepsy will be controlled and outgrown. It would be a pity if anxiety and overprotection left your child truly handicapped. To achieve a full and normal life you and your child must both become active, informed, optimistic participants. We hope that this book has helped, and that your child will live a healthy, full, seizure-free life.

# Glossary

**Absence seizure**  A generalized seizure in which consciousness is altered, formerly called "petit mal," a term now seldom used. It is usually brief; similar seizures occur many times in a day. The EEG pattern is three per second spikes and waves. Absence seizures are usually easily treated and usually outgrown.

**Ambulatory monitoring**  The use of a cassette-like tape recorder to monitor the EEG while an individual is up, around, at work, school, or play. The ambulatory monitoring device permits up to twenty-four hours of recording on tape. However, the amount of information produced about specific parts of the brain is limited. Since either the child or another observer must mark events thought to be seizures, and because the amount of EEG information is limited, ambulatory monitoring is useful only in special situations where it is important to clarify the nature of the spell (i.e., faint vs seizure) and where quantification of spells is important. Far less expensive than video-EEG monitoring, but also less definitive.

**Anticonvulsant**  One of the drugs used to prevent recurrence of seizures. The particular drug chosen for a child depends on the type of seizures, the age of the child, and the type of side effect that might be expected.

**Association cortex**  The part of the brain in the parietal lobe where vision, hearing, memories, and motor function come together and where associations occur between sensations, movements, and thoughts.

**Atonic seizures**  A form of generalized seizure in which body tone is suddenly lost and the child slumps to the ground or his head slumps forward. These difficult-to-control seizures often occur in the Lennox-Gastaut syndrome. They may resemble the sudden seizure in which the child is thrown to the ground, often injuring his face or teeth.

| | |
|---|---|
| | This more forceful seizure is a type of myoclonic seizure. |
| **Atypical absence** | Staring spell similar to absence seizures, but often with an "atypical" EEG. It may last longer than the typical absence seizure and may have other additional features (movement, falling, etc.). Atypical absence may be more difficult to control with medications than typical absence seizures. |
| **Aura** | The start of a seizure. It is usually described as a warning—a peculiar feeling, a sense of fear, a funny sensation in one part of the body. This activity can spread to other areas of the brain. If the seizure does not spread, the aura would also be referred to as a simple partial seizure. |
| **Automatisms** | The complex and purposeless automatic movements that accompany a complex partial seizure. These movements often consist of smacking of the lips, chewing, picking at clothes, or wandering around in a confused fashion. |
| **Autonomic** | The autonomic nervous system is the part of the brain that controls functions like heart rate, blood pressure, skin temperature, and color. Seizures from the temporal lobe can produce disturbances of autonomic function. |
| **Axon** | The part of a neuron that resembles a telephone line in that it is responsible for the capacity to communicate with another cell. |
| **Benign rolandic epilepsy** | A special form of seizures in children starting after three years of age. The seizure often starts with a sensation in the corner of the mouth, followed by local jerking of the muscles; it spreads to one side of the face, or one side of the body, and may become a generalized seizure. It has a typical EEG. These seizures occur more commonly during certain stages of sleep. They are usually outgrown. |
| **Breathholding spell** | An episode in which the child does not breathe, turns blue, and may lose consciousness. These spells may, on occasion, result in a seizure. Breathholding spells are not serious and are not epilepsy. There are two forms: cyanotic (blue) and pallid (white). |
| **Clonic seizure** | The rhythmic jerking of an extremity or the whole body. Clonic seizures are rare. They are the |

|                          | second component of tonic-clonic seizures and seldom occur without a preceding tonic phase. |
|--------------------------|--------------------------------------------------------------------------------------------|
| **Complex partial seizure** | A seizure that involves only part of the brain (usually the temporal or the frontal lobe) *and* that alters consciousness or awareness. It may be accompanied by automatisms. "Complex partial seizures" and "partial complex seizures" mean the same thing. |
| **Consciousness** | Alertness or awareness, the ability to interact normally with the environment. Consciousness is altered in generalized seizures or complex partial seizures, but is usually not affected in simple partial seizures. |
| **Convulsion** | An older term for a seizure. It usually refers to seizures that have a motor component—jerking or stiffening. Other old terms for convulsion include "spell" or "fit." |
| **Convulsive syncope** | A seizure that occurs in association with a fainting spell. The child experiences sweatiness, pallor, dizziness, and faints and loses consciousness. A small percentage of people who faint will then have a brief tonic-clonic seizure. The fainting spell is termed syncope; when a tonic-clonic seizure is associated with it, it is called convulsive syncope. The convulsion of convulsive syncope is a benign seizure and does not require treatment. |
| **CT scan** | CT scan, or CAT scan, uses small doses of x-rays and computer analysis to produce a picture of the brain and allow the physician to see certain abnormalities. |
| **Cyanotic breathholding spells** | Breathholding spells in which the child starts to cry, then holds his breath and turns blue before losing consciousness. A seizure occasionally follows a breathholding spell. |
| **Cysticerosis** | An infection of the brain in which cysts within the brain become calcified and cause seizures. It is more common in underdeveloped than in developed countries. |
| **Déjà vu** | A sensation that you have seen something or someone before, whether or not you have. This sensation is normal and common, but when it occurs repeatedly, it can be a manifestation of complex partial seizures emanating from the temporal lobe. |

| | |
|---|---|
| **EEG** (electroencephalogram) | Recording of the electrical activity or "brain waves" of the brain. The EEG does not provide a diagnosis of epilepsy, but it assists physicians in clarifying the type or origin of seizures. |
| **Encephalitis** | Inflammation of the brain substance itself, due to bacterial or viral infection. |
| **Epilepsies, The** | Seizure patterns whose clinical manifestations and EEGs are sufficiently characteristic for a physician to be able to predict a patient's future course and to recommend specific medications. The term "the epilepsies" is also used to indicate that there are diverse forms of repeated seizures (epilepsy), not just one single type. |
| **Epilepsy** | Recurrent (two or more) seizures not provoked by specific events such as trauma, infection, fever, or chemical changes. Seizures may take many forms. Patterns of epilepsy that are similar and have a predictable outcome are termed epileptic syndromes. |
| **Epileptic cephalalgia** | The headache that follows some seizures. Seizures increase blood flow to the brain; resulting dilation of blood vessels may cause a post-seizure headache. Migraine headaches can be mistaken for epileptic cephalalgia. |
| **Epileptic syndrome** | A pattern that includes seizure type, age at onset, characteristic EEG, and an expected outcome. Certain epileptic syndromes respond better to particular types of medications. Epileptic syndromes include infantile spasms, the Lennox-Gastaut syndrome, benign rolandic epilepsy, and others. The various epileptic syndromes make up the epilepsies. |
| **Epileptogenic** | Susceptible to a seizure. Areas of the brain more susceptible to seizures than other areas are considered epileptogenic. The temporal and frontal lobes are usually more epileptogenic than other regions. |
| **Febrile seizure** | A seizure caused by fever. Febrile seizures are common in young children, of six months to three or four years old. Resulting from a low threshold of the young brain, only rarely are they associated with later epilepsy. While frightening, they appear to cause little harm. They tend to occur in families. Physicians generally do not prescribe anticonvulsants to try to prevent these seizures. |

| | |
|---|---|
| Fit | A term still often used in England to refer to a seizure. Most other physicians prefer to avoid using that term to describe seizure episodes. |
| Focal resection | Surgical removal of one area or region of the brain. |
| Focal seizures | See simple partial seizures. |
| Focus | A local area of abnormality in the brain. These local abnormalities may be seen as spikes, or sharp waves, or as slowing on an EEG. |
| Generalized seizure | A seizure involving the whole brain. It may involve alterations of alertness or awareness, as during absence or complex partial seizures, or tonic-clonic movements of both sides of the body. |
| Grand mal | The old term for generalized tonic-clonic seizures. |
| Hemispherectomy | Surgical removal of one-half of the brain. There are several different types of hemispherectomy performed. |
| History | The detailed medical story of previous events. The history establishes exactly what happened to the patient and explores the general state of a person's health. |
| Hyperventilate | To over-breathe. A physician may instruct your child to take a number of deep breathes for two to four minutes. This over-ventilation may cause an absence or complex partial seizure, which can then be observed by your doctor. Rapid breathing during exercise is rarely associated with a seizure. Anxiety may cause an individual to over-breathe or to hyperventilate. |
| Hypsarrhythmia | A term used to describe the EEG frequently seen in children who have had infantile spasms. This characteristic EEG pattern is wildly chaotic, of very high voltage, with many spikes and slow waves. The terms hypsarrhythmia and infantile spasm are often, although incorrectly, used interchangeably. |
| Ictal (Ictus) | A Latin term for "stroke" or "event." A seizure, of whatever type, is referred to as an ictus. |
| Idiopathic | Of unknown cause. Seizures are called "idiopathic seizures" if no cause can be found. Causes cannot be found in more than half of the children experiencing seizures. Idiopathic seizures often have a better outcome than those that are "symptomatic," that is, for which a cause can be found. |
| Infantile spasms | A special form of epilepsy in the first two years of life with multiple causes. The seizures consist of |

repeated episodes of flexion of the head on the chest, the knees coming up, and the arms extending. Each episode lasts one to two seconds; episodes occur in a series of five to fifty, with a brief pause between each. The child may have many such series during each day. This form of epilepsy is commonly associated with significant mental retardation and requires prompt diagnosis and treatment with specific medication to try to halt the process.

**Intensive monitoring**    Monitoring, using modern technology, of the characteristics of an individual's seizures and their correlation with an EEG. Monitoring may include ambulatory monitoring, prolonged EEGs, prolonged video-EEG monitoring, and use of depth electrodes and the grid.

**Inter-ictal**    The period between episodes or seizures. (*See* Ictal.)

**Janz, juvenile myoclonic epilepsy of ("JME")**    A newly recognized syndrome that begins in late childhood with mild myoclonic jerks on going to sleep or awakening. This jerking may precede or be associated with absence seizures or generalized tonic-clonic seizures. It is often produced by sleep deprivation and commonly runs in families. The characteristic EEG and history make diagnosis of this condition easy, and treatment is usually very effective.

**Lennox-Gastaut syndrome**    A condition that includes two or more types of seizures, one of which is of the akinetic, atonic, falling-down type. Absence seizures and generalized tonic-clonic seizures, occurring particularly at night, are common. The EEG shows generalized slow spike or poly-spike and slow wave abnormalities. Mental retardation is common and often progressive. This is a severe seizure type and one that is difficult to control.

**Lobes**    Functional parts of the brain. The principal lobes include the frontal lobes, important for personality and memory; the temporal lobes, which are responsible for speech, memory,and emotion; the parietal lobes, which integrate sensory function; and the occipital lobes, which are the site of vision.

**Meningitis**    Inflammation of the coverings of the brain caused by bacteria or viral infections. Meningitis may be accompanied by inflammation of the brain itself (encephalitis), resulting on occasion in seizures or brain damage.

| | |
|---|---|
| **Migraine** | Migraine headaches, caused by changes within the blood vessels of the brain, are characteristically accompanied by paleness, nausea, vomiting, and sleep. They often last more than an hour. On rare occasions they can be confused with or associated with seizures. They tend to run in families. |
| **Minor motor seizure** | An old term, not part of the new classification, previously used to describe multiple types of spells, including atonic and myoclonic varieties. Children with the Lennox-Gastaut syndrome generally experience multiple types of seizures, many of which are "minor motor." |
| **MRI scan** | Magnetic resonance imaging scans, like CT scans, are used to identify structure and abnormalities within the brain. This new technique uses no x-ray and gives a clearer picture of brain structure than does the CT scan. It is more expensive and takes longer to do than the CT scan. |
| **Myoclonic jerks** | Sudden movements of arms or legs, most commonly occurring when the child is falling asleep. Myoclonic jerks during the day may be normal, but if frequent could be part of one of the epilepsies. |
| **Myoclonic seizures** | Sudden jerks of muscle groups that resemble sudden jolts "like an electric shock." These jerks may be of a hand, a leg, a shoulder, or sudden flexion of the body forward or backward. While occasional myoclonic jerks may be normal, repeated myoclonic jerks can be a difficult-to-control form of epilepsy. |
| **Neurofibromatosis** | An inherited condition characterized by brown (*cafe-au-lait* or coffee-colored) spots, mild mental retardation, and seizures. Small tumors on many nerves may compress surrounding tissue causing pain, weakness, etc. |
| **Neurons** | The nerve cells of the brain. |
| **Neurotransmitter** | The chemicals released by the ending (terminal) of an axon that float across the space between cells and affect the "firing" of the next cell. Neurotransmitters may be excitatory or inhibitory to the next cell. |
| **Pallid breathholding spells** | Not true breathholding, but a sudden loss of consciousness due to slowing of the heart, usu- |

ally occurring after mild trauma. They may, on occasion, result in a seizure. They are not epilepsy and rarely require treatment.

**Partial complex seizures**    Another name for complex partial seizures.

**Partial seizures**    Partial seizures are focal or local seizures in the brain.

**Petit mal**    The old term for "little spells" now known as "absence" seizures. These "little spells" usually include staring. Many kinds of seizures include staring and respond to different medications.

**Photic sensitive seizure**    Seizure caused by flashing lights, such as strobe lights or light shining through trees or a fence. In some "photic sensitive" individuals these stimuli may produce seizures.

**Post-ictal**    A Latin term meaning after the seizure (see ictus). Confusion, sleepiness, or weakness after the seizure is termed post-ictal since it occurs after the event.

**Prognosis**    Outcome or outlook of a medical condition. For certain types of seizures, and certain epilepsies, the "prognosis" can be predicted.

**Pseudo-seizures**    Events that resemble seizures but are not caused, as a seizure is, by electrical abnormalities in the brain. Pseudo-seizures may be a child's conscious imitation of seizures, a way of coping with stress, or may be subconscious. Pseudo-seizures often occur in persons who also have true seizures and may be difficult to differentiate from true seizures.

**Rasmussen's syndrome**    A rare, progressive, condition that is characterized by unilateral seizures and progressive one-sided paralysis. Of unknown cause, this condition is best treated with hemispherectomy.

**Recruitment**    In physiologic terms, or in regard to epilepsy, recruitment refers to an enlisting of surrounding cells to fire simultaneously. Only when a certain number of cells are recruited to fire together will sufficient electrical activity be generated to appear as a spike on the EEG or as a clinical seizure.

**Seizure**    A paroxysmal (episodic) electrical discharge of neurons (nerve cells) in the brain resulting in alteration of function or behavior. There are many different forms of seizures, depending on where in the brain the electrical activity starts and on the direction and rapidity of its spread in the brain.

**Simple partial seizures**  Focal or local seizures involving a single area of the brain. Since the region involved has particular functions, there are many kinds of simple partial seizures depending on which region is affected. Some are motor, involving the face, hand, or leg; some sensory, with individual sensations in a part of the body; some involving a temporal lobe, producing smells, tastes, fears, or memories. Unlike a complex partial seizure, consciousness is not altered in a simple partial seizure.

**Sleep myoclonus**  Sudden massive jerks of the body, as when someone is going to sleep, are normal. They are termed "sleep myoclonus."

**Spell**  A term used to describe seizures. The term is vague and is often used to refer to a seizure or a pseudo-seizure if the nature of that episode is unknown.

**Spike**  A sharp abnormality appearing on the EEG that indicates an electrical discharge of a small number of neighboring brain cells. Recurrent spikes are electrical seizures and may spread to involve sufficient brain cells to cause a true change in function or behavior, that is, a clinical seizure.

**Storage diseases**  Multiple metabolic diseases in which some material, usually a breakdown product of normal tissue, cannot be further metabolized and is stored within nerve cells of the brain. This storage produces malfunction of the cells; it is commonly associated with progressive intellectual and neurologic deterioration and with seizures. Each of the various diseases has a name.

**Sturge-Weber disease**  A disease, characterized by a birthmark (hemangioma or port wine stain) involving the forehead and variable parts of the face, often associated with vascular abnormality of the brain, seizures, progressive one-sided weakness, and progressive mental retardation.

**Symptomatic**  Refers to a defined cause. Seizures due to fever, meningitis, chemical abnormalities, or head trauma are called "symptomatic seizures" or provoked seizures.

| | |
|---|---|
| Synapse | The tiny space between the ending of the axon and the body of the next neuron. |
| Syncope | Fainting. The characteristics include a feeling of dizziness associated with pallor and sweatiness, followed by loss of consciousness. When this benign condition is followed by a brief tonic-clonic seizure, it is termed "convulsive syncope." |
| Syndrome | A collection of signs or symptoms that together form a condition with a known outcome, or which requires special treatment. |
| Threshold | The susceptibility of a single neuron to fire or of the brain to have a seizure. Many factors may lower the brain threshold and precipitate a seizure. Anticonvulsant drugs raise the threshold and make seizures less likely. |
| Tics | A sudden, episodic, repetitive movement, most commonly involving eye-blinking or movements of the face and head, but sometimes other parts of the body. These complex movements are not associated with alterations in consciousness, and they can usually be stopped consciously for periods of time. They are not associated with EEG abnormalities and are not seizures. |
| Todd's paralysis | Weakness occurring in one limb or one side of the body after a focal or unilateral seizure. This paralysis, while often thought of as exhaustion of the brain, actually results from inhibition of the seizures and of the normal function of the brain on that side. Todd's paralysis after a seizure is usually resolved in one to two hours but may, on occasion, continue for several days. It always recovers completely. |
| Tonic-clonic seizures | Generalized seizures people often think of when they think of epilepsy, formerly called "grand mal" seizures. They are associated with stiffening and then rhythmic jerking movements of the body. |
| Tonic seizures | In a tonic seizure a child stiffens her arms, legs, and back (becomes tonic) and loses consciousness; the stiffening may last several seconds to a minute. Most tonic seizures go on to a clonic component. Tonic seizures are uncommon, except as the first part of the tonic-clonic seizure. |
| Toxoplasmosis | A chronic infection often acquired by a fetus *in utero* that affects multiple organ systems. It can |

cause mental retardation, scarring of the brain, and seizures.

**Tuberous sclerosis**    A disease characterized by skin lesions (white spots, thickened patches, etc.), seizures, and mental retardation. Because it is caused by abnormal development of cells, many other organs of the body (e.g., leg, heart, kidneys) experience changes or tumors.

**Unilateral seizure**    A seizure involving one side of the body, usually the face, arm, or leg. A unilateral seizure involves or spreads through a single half of the brain.

**Video-EEG**    The use of video cameras to capture visually the onset and characteristics of seizures or episodes while simultaneously monitoring the EEG to see electrical changes. Video-EEG monitoring permits a physician to identify whether a seizure is associated with an EEG change, that is, real or a pseudo-seizure. It will often allow physicians to identify areas in the brain where the seizures begin.

# Index

Absence seizures, 62–63, 92, 93(fig.); atypical, 92; coping with, 186–88
Acceptance, 181, 197, 234
ACTH. *See* Adrenocorticotropic hormone
Adrenocorticotropic hormone, as treatment for infantile spasms, 109–10
Age, seizures and, 17(fig.)
AIDS, 115
Allergic reactions, to drugs, 131
Ambulance, when to call, 54
Ambulatory EEG monitoring. *See* Electroencephalogram, ambulatory
Amygdala, 72, 73(fig.)
Anticonvulsant drugs; blood levels and therapeutic range of, 124–30; breastfeeding and, 264; and diagnosis of seizures, 23; discontinuing, 139, 146–49; how they work, 120–24; paroxysmal behavior disturbances and, 33; pregnancy and, 260–63; risks and benefits of, 46–51
Antiepileptic drugs, pharmacological facts, 125(table)
Anxiety, 197. *See also* Epilepsy, coping with
Ataxia, drugs and, 121
Ativan. *See* Lorazepam
Atonic seizures, 64
Attention problems, 242–44
Auras: migraine headaches and, 32–33; as phase of seizure, 59
Automatisms, 73
Autonomic functions, area of brain, 72
Autonomic symptoms, simple partial seizures with, 76
Axons, interconnection of neurons, 12, 13(fig.)

Behavior, epilepsy and, 239–48
Behavioral disturbances, paroxysmal, 33
Benign rolandic epilepsy, 106–7
Bike riding, risks of, 51
Birth control pills, 264
Blood count, carbamazepine and, 134
Brain: anatomy of, 66–76(figs.); degenera-

tive diseases of, 116; development abnormalities in, 112–16
Breastfeeding, anticonvulsant drugs and, 264
Breathholding spells, 30–31

Calcium, 151
Carbamazepine, 134, 125(table); side effects of, 134–36
Cerebral palsy, seizures and, 203–6
Chemical changes, seizures and, 17–18(fig.)
Clonazepam, 138
Clorazepate, 138
Colic, infantile spasms mistaken for, 108
Computerized tomography (CT), 102–5, 112
Concussion, seizures and, 24
Corpus callosum, sectioning, 169–70
Counseling, 220–36

Daydreaming, seizures and, 28–29
Decision-making, 46–50
Déjà vu, area of brain, 72
Depakene. *See* Valproic acid
Depakote. *See* Valproic acid
Depression, 219
Depth electrodes, invasive studies for epilepsy, 164
Diazepam, 138
Diet, and epilepsy, 150–55. *See also* Ketogenic diet
Dilantin. *See* Phenytoin
Diplegia, 205
Disability, seizures and, 189
Driving, risks of, 255–58
Drug levels, 121; allergic reactions, 131. *See also* Anticonvulsant drugs
Drugs: generic, 139; therapeutic ranges of, 124–30; toxicity of, 121

EEG. *See* Electroencephalogram
Electroencephalogram: ambulatory, 98–99; brain activity during, 87–95(figs.); intensive monitoring with, 97; interactions in brain, 10; specialized pro-

Design by Kachergis Book Design
Composed by The Composing Room of Michigan, Inc. in Sabon
text and Helvetica display
Printed by R.R. Donnelley & Sons Company on 50-lb. Sebago
Cream White paper